Clinical Teaching in Nursing

Clinical Teaching in Nursing

Ruth White
Visiting Fellow
School of Medical Education
University of New South Wales
Australia

and

Christine Ewan
Professor and Dean
Faculty of Health and
Behavioural Sciences
University of Wollongong
Australia

SPRINGER-SCIENCE+BUSINESS MEDIA, B.V.

First edition 1991

Originally published by Chapman & Hall in 1991
MyCopy version of the original edition 1991

Typeset in 10/12 pt Palatino by Best-set Typesetter Ltd, Hong Kong

DOI 10.1007/978-1-4899-3354-6

A catalogue record for this book is available from the British Library

Library of Congress Cataloging-in-Publication data
White, Ruth, 1926–
Clinical teaching in nursing / Ruth White and Christine Ewan.—
1st ed.
p. cm.
Companion v. to: Teaching nursing / Christine Ewan and Ruth White. c1984.
Includes bibliographical references and index.
1. Nursing—Study and teaching. I. Ewan, Christine E.
II. Ewan, Christine E. Teaching nursing III. Title.
[DNLM: 1 Clinical Competence. 2. Education, Nursing.
3. Teaching—methods. WY 18 W587c]
RT90.W55 1991
610.73'07—dc20
DNLM/DLC
for Library of Congress 91–20220
www.springer.com/mycopy CIP

Contents

Preface

This book aims to assist clinical teachers in the practice of clinical teaching. It assumes that clinical teachers will bring to their task a background knowledge of educational principles, experience in a clinical nursing field, knowledge of substantive nursing content, a love of teaching and a desire to share with their students the joys, tears, challenge and wonder of learning in the clinical setting. The format is designed around a set of commonly encountered problems and encourages readers, whether on the threshold of a career as a clinical teacher or those who are experienced, to think through their responses to the problem situation before reading on to a disclosure of possible courses of action.

In brief, the book is a companion to *Teaching Nursing: A Self-Instructional Handbook* (Ewan and White, 1984).

The authors' interest in clinical teaching can be traced through a number of years in a variety of teaching careers with multidisciplinary health professional groups, of whom nurses comprise the majority of practitioners. As senior lecturers in the School of Medical Education, the authors were involved in developing and teaching a Master of Health Personnel Education Degree course; the students (or Fellows) in that programme were all graduates from a broad range of health care disciplines – nursing, medicine, physiotherapy, occupational therapy, nutrition, dentistry, health education, health resources management, radiography, social work, community development, occupational safety and health. Issues of clinical teaching were raised both during course work and also, more searchingly, by Fellows who chose a clinical education problem as the focus of the research project component of the degree (Higgs, 1982; Ritchie, 1986; Lumby, 1987; Tan, 1987; Kermode, 1987; Mill, 1989; Pratt, 1989; Sando, 1989).

Both authors have been involved in research projects in clinical teaching which involved observational study of clinical teaching, interviews with students and teachers and development of video-taped clinical teaching scenarios for use in clinical teaching in nursing, medicine and physiotherapy. The research indicated that some commonly held assumptions about clinical teaching needed to be challenged. Assumptions such as the following were not borne out by our observations of clinical teaching:

1. Being an effective lecturer in the lecture hall or classroom guarantees effective teaching in a clinical setting.
2. Being an expert clinician ensures that a person would also be an expert clinical teacher.
3. Clinical teaching skills are no different from classroom teaching skills.

Funding was obtained from the Clive and Vera Ramaciotti Foundations for a two-year project to develop a series of videotaped segments on clinical teaching microskills.* During that project, observations of clinical teaching and interviews with clinical teachers revealed that most programmes in nursing had adopted a pattern of systematic progression through the presentation of theory, laboratory practice, briefing or preconference before clinical practice and debriefing or post-conference after clinical practice. Some programmes added a further component to obtain feedback on all stages of 'the clinical learning cycle' from teachers and students involved.

While it is true that the briefing and debriefing segments of the cycle appear in many fields of education, and that extensive exploration of their use has been documented (Goldhammer, 1969; Matheney, 1969; Turney *et al.*, 1982; Schon, 1988; Boud, *et al.*, 1985; Boud, 1988; Smyth, 1984, 1986) the full cycle of learning has important implications for clinical teachers in nursing. Whereas, in the past, students were expected to take from theory what was required for practice without intermediary learning stages and preparation for practice, the cycle offered a logical progression for students and teachers and a close link of theory with practice. The clinical learning cycle provides the framework of the book.

A second project, funded in 1988 by the Bicentennial Foundation,

* *Positive Practices. Microskills for clinical teachers in nurse education.* Audio Visual Unit, University of New South Wales, Sydney.

Teaching Practices. Microskills for teachers in medical education and the therapies. Audio Visual Unit, University of New South Wales, Sydney.

through the Committee to Review Australian Studies in Tertiary Education, enabled the production of a set of taped programmes.* This project aimed to provide examples of ways the clinical teacher could include social and behavioural science perspectives in clinical teaching. The assumption was that the application of biological sciences has certain universal similarities, but that the social context is culturally, locally and often individually bound. There are fewer models of application to follow than in the biological or physical sciences. The Bicentennial project sought to identify Australian material appropriate to each critical incident in nursing.

This book draws on some of the material and observations gained during those two projects and the contribution of staff and students in Health Professional Schools is acknowledged with warm appreciation.

* *Critical Incidents in Clinical Teaching. Perspectives from the Social and Behavioural Sciences*. Audio Visual Unit, University of New South Wales, Sydney.

1

Clinical teaching

Students have little hesitation in telling us what does and what does not help them to learn in clinical settings. Repeatedly, student evaluations of their clinical learning experience leave teachers in no doubt that their involvement with students, the support they give, the confidence they can engender, the clinical expertise they model and the knowledge they share, are important to students' clinical learning (Windsor, 1987). Clinical teachers express a need for guidance in assisting students to apply their own knowledge to problems in practice that are real and individual. Teachers also know that what students are seeing and doing in clinical work can often remain at a superficial level of practice unless they are stimulated to analyse and synthesize their observations and to question the meaning of their experience and its implications for future experiences. In this respect clinical teaching is so far removed from classroom teaching that teachers confronted by the complexity of the task are often bewildered and anxious, or alternatively, paralysed into inactivity and passive supervision.

This chapter defines clinical teaching, the environment in which it is practised, the role of the clinical teacher and the challenges facing clinical teaching today. It also sketches the framework for analysis of clinical teaching upon which the rest of the book is based.

1.1 WHAT IS CLINICAL TEACHING?

Although 'clinical' usually carries the connotation of the 'sick-bed' (from *clinikos* = bed), the term is also applied to teaching in fields other than the health professions. Most notably, in teacher education, where the 'clinical approach' in the educational supervision of learner-teachers was adopted in the 1950s. The intent was 'to describe a form of professional learning that endorses the primacy of the patient/client/pupil and the situational context in which this occurs' (Smyth, 1986, p. 2). Interestingly, the situational context for clinical teaching in nursing is just as likely to be non-institutional and health-related as it is to be focused around the 'sick-bed'. In this text, clinical teaching will be assumed to take place in any context in which teacher, client and student have face-to-face contact. There will be additional occasions when the client is not present, but is, nevertheless, the focus of the learning and teaching; these occasions will also be designated as clinical teaching.

Although there are many ways of expressing what clinical teaching is, definitions usually contain some reference to the translation of basic theoretical knowledge into practice. Schweer (1972) calls it the 'vehicle that provides students with the opportunity to translate basic theoretical knowledge into the learning of a variety of intellectual and psychomotor skills needed to provide patient-centred quality nursing care' (p. 41). A more comprehensive definition includes additional steps before and after the transfer of basic principles into clinical performance. According to Meleca *et al.* (1978) clinical teaching is

> preparing students to integrate previously acquired basic science information with performance-oriented skills and competencies associated with the diagnosis, treatment, and care of patients and to acquire the kinds of professional and personal skills, attitudes and behaviours thought essential for entering the health care system and embarking on continuing forms of education.

Benner (1989) points out that there is another important dimension in clinical teaching, that is, the uncovering of the 'complexity and richness of the practice we want to teach' (p. 25). In other words, clinical teaching, in its focus on the relationship between theory and practice, can assist students to not only apply theory, but also to search the ways that nursing theory can emerge from the rich texture of clinical practice.

The literature has much to offer in consideration of the influences of technical, practical and critical approaches to thinking and action (Carr and Kemmis, 1986). In the definitions of clinical teaching it is possible to trace all three approaches. In later chapters implications of choosing a technical, practical or critical approach to clinical teaching and learning will be included where appropriate.

1.2 THE ENVIRONMENT FOR CLINICAL TEACHING AND LEARNING

The skills of the clinical teacher during the clinical practice session are critical. Different types of skill will be called for, depending on the level of the students, the demands of the situation and importantly, the educational philosophy of the teacher. Over-riding all the considerations the clinical teacher can bring to the task, however, is the environment in which the student, the teacher and the client find themselves. Engaged in a teaching session, each will be affected differently; each will respond differently. The clinical teacher's responsibility is to prepare all three participants for the session and to observe sensitively during the session for unanticipated environmental complexities.

Complexities of the setting

Although the impact of the complexity of the setting of clinical practice on the practitioner has often been taken for granted (and until recently not considered an important area of investigation), the effect on the learner and the client has rated even less consideration. In contrast with the controlled environment of the lecture hall with its large, usually anonymous classes addressed by a lecturer with the aid of a microphone, the environment of the clinical teacher and students is unpredictable, volatile, dynamic, close and personal.

Without doubt, the presence of the patient makes clinical teaching a powerful centre for learning. For the teacher, attempting to capitalize on the experience for students, the planning task is daunting. A classroom session can be planned to take account of relevance, meaningfulness and sequence, in the knowledge that the conditions for teaching will remain static. This is not so in a clinical teaching session. A session planned to meet certain objectives may have to be abandoned at short notice because of sudden changes in the patient or the clinical setting. Mastering each segment of the course of study presents no problem for the classroom teacher and the continuity of the teaching topic can be ensured. On the other hand, knowing each patient's history and being aware of the events in his/her treatment and progress may not be possible in advance of a clinical teaching session.

Although students are learners rather than employees they are also involved in the occupational pattern of nursing in an institution. Often the tasks, schedules and routines take precedence over the learning objectives. The clinical teacher is faced with a dilemma; students need to be prepared for the 'real world' of work while also distinguishing between effective and not so effective work schedules. The aim of clinical nursing practice is patient care and administrative efficiency; in clinical learning and teaching the aim is educative. While the distinction appears to be clear, there is, in reality a very fine line between the nursing task to be done and the learning of students during that task. This may appear to be a pedantic distinction, but the need to identify clearly what the student is learning, while also doing, also has industrial implications, as was highlighted in a legal battle in Australia in 1988 (The Registered Nurses Professional Rates Case, No. 2. 1988). The clinical teacher and students must appreciate the distinction and work within it.

Examined more closely, the environment for clinical teaching challenges the most imaginative teachers. The real, as compared to the theoretical, situation imposes emotional demands. Many distractions are present and compete for the student's attention. The complexities of dealing with the unpleasant (sights, smells, cries of pain) and the difficult problems (an abusive or disturbed person) impinge on the learner, teacher and patient. Viewed from the safety and distance of the classroom, clinical problems are amenable to cognitive solutions; in the reality of the clinical setting each problem becomes immediately charged with personal responses. Values and ethics, as well as practical, affective and cognitive issues are involved. How does this affect learning? What can the teacher do?

The clinical learning environment

Such a variety of challenges presents a different mental set for students and teachers than is common in the classroom. Few curricula are designed to integrate subject matter around clinical problems or concepts. When students study separate subjects, each with an intrinsic disciplinary structure, there is a problem in applying relevant information to individual clinical problems. For example, there is no separation of a person's physiology from his or her psychology, ethnicity or socio-economic status. Students need guidance, therefore, in applying theoretical material, not as separate subjects, but interwoven.

In the classroom, using reading material and problem-solving exercises as resources, the ideal clinical answer to a patient's problem can be obtained. In the clinical setting, with the client as the resource, the real and possible answer to the person's problem in the midst of the complexities of the clinical environment often presents a conflict for students as they try to reconcile the ideal with the real.

It is no longer sufficient to plan simply for a period of 'time spent' in a clinical area. Achievement of explicit learning objectives as specified by the curriculum, as well as clinical objectives is demanded. In addition, students need to learn how to set their own personal learning objectives. The potency of clinical settings requires that clinical teachers know how to channel the students' readiness to learn into achievable and realistic outcomes.

For students, the differences between learning in the classroom and in clinical are profound. The anonymity of many classrooms shields the students from the teacher's close attention. In the clinical setting, in a small group, students are known and can feel threatened. They are certainly vulnerable. Teachers have more frequent direct access to evidence of students' performance and while students want realistic feedback, they also fear the teacher's dual role of teacher and assessor. Achievement of cognitive objectives and evidence of cognitive mastery is rewarded in the classroom; attitudinal and practical skills as well as intellectual skills are required in clinical. The complexity of the clinical environment, the pressures of the clinical learning task and the demands of interacting appropriately with both teacher and patient, prescribe for students a set of circumstances in which they must learn to acquire professional performance skills.

It is taken for granted that students learn clinical skills 'by doing' but this assumption has probably been responsible for the not uncommon belief that clinical learning is automatic, or 'habit' learning and that clinical teaching is, therefore, a less demanding task than classroom teaching. There has certainly been a paucity of research in clinical teaching. In comparison with the number of texts on research based classroom teaching (Turney *et al.*, 1982), research based books on clinical teaching in nursing are rare with a few notable exceptions such as Infante's text (1975, revised 1985), which is based on her doctoral research. Other doctoral studies have researched clinical teaching problems (for example, Carr, 1983; Chuaprapaisilp, 1989) but their studies have not been published as texts.

Learning from experience is not the simple 'learning by doing' which has been accepted in the past. Accounts of the learning potential of experience (Dewey, 1983; Kolb, 1984; Boud, 1988) illuminate the nature of clinical learning, and mandate a re-examination of what students can gain from their experience. A more detailed discussion of experiential learning is given in Chapter 2.

Clinical learning in a community environment

With earlier discharge of clients, demands for nursing in the community have increased. Students are inexperienced, and require teaching, assistance and supervision in community practice settings. Clinical teachers themselves need to be informed not only about the patient's history and condition, but about the student's level of learning and experience in community nursing.

The one-to-one emphasis of practice in the institutional setting may not be as appropriate for community practice where the families and support networks of individual clients are also the focus of community health nursing. Teaching health practices to a group in a health centre calls for specialized skills, very different from the individualized health teaching necessary for clients during hospital care and prior to discharge. The emphasis on health promotion, prevention as well as cure, gives to students a perception of continuity of practice not always possible in the institution. The climate for teaching and learning in the community opens another world for the student where wellness, rather than illness is the focus.

The relative freedom of the community setting and in particular, the position of the teacher and student as visitors in the client's own home, casts the teaching/learning triad of teacher, student and client within the client's, not the health professionals', culture. Questions of life styles, values, health priorities, acceptance or rejection of care and counsel by the client, could challenge the student's sensitivity to the complex forces that influence health care decisions (Reilly and Oermann, 1985). In response to the influences of the community on teaching, the clinical teacher's primary function is in preparing students for working in the ambiguity of a relatively unstructured milieu.

1.3 IMPLICATIONS OF THE CLINICAL LEARNING ENVIRONMENT

Control of the learning session

In many nursing programmes the clinical teacher is also a classroom teacher and moves with the students throughout the theoretical, laboratory, pre- and post-conference phases as well as clinical practice. Other programmes assign clinical teachers to teach students in clinical practice sessions only. Whatever the system adopted by an educational institution, the environment for clinical teaching and learning exerts lifelong influences on both teacher and students. Some of the shared experiences with patients will be poignant and unforgettable; some alarming and frightening; others humdrum. Because of the variety of experiences, it follows that students will not achieve identical clinical learning. There is little point, therefore, in trying to control the learning environment and provide common experience, as would be the case in the classroom. Control of experiences in each session is unlikely to be possible, and in fact, is likely to be highly undesirable. The unplanned, unpredictable events are learning moments which can be capitalized on by a teacher who is alert to identify for students observations and insights they would otherwise not recognize themselves.

The roles of the clinical teacher

Most clinical teachers will agree that they play many roles during the phases of clinical teaching in lab, briefing and debriefing as well as in the clinical/community setting. They will also agree that they often take multiple roles within a single clinical teaching episode. The teaching role can expand to include, for example such roles as counsellor, problem solver, manager, assessor, advocate, guide and facilitator. Infante (1975) in the first edition of her text points to the role of the clinical teacher as it relates to the activities of the student in the clinical setting in this way:

> the emphasis in the clinical laboratory should not be on how to care, but on how to apply knowledges to care for clients. Caring is not synonymous with learning (p. 23).

The inference Infante draws from this is that the role of the teacher should be clearly stated to reflect the use of the clinical laboratory,

> when the student needs to see and cope with these real-life situations and learns to apply knowledge to practice in order to render care (p. 24).

In the 1985 edition of her text, Infante is emphatic about what the student as learner is doing in the clinical setting while the role of the teacher is one of orchestration of relevant student activities.

> The teacher does not teach in the clinical laboratory. The teaching has been done before the use of the clinical laboratory, that is, in the classroom and college laboratory. Relevant activities are orchestrated by the teacher for the student to experience in his or her own fashion. The clinical laboratory is the culminating activity that affords the student the opportunity to practise already acquired intellectual and psychomotor skills – not to acquire the theoretical principles behind the skills (p. 5).

The role of the clinical teacher as guide, facilitator and supporter during a clinical learning session is the model proposed in this book. The skills required in the role are further developed in later chapters and are dependent on the successful implementation of college laboratory, and pre-clinical or briefing sessions, each requiring additional and different skills. The debriefing or post-conference session completes the clinical learning cycle which also demands specific clinical teaching skills.

Stevens (1979) focuses clinical teaching within a framework of 'education for practical activity' (p. 161). The role of the clinical teacher is to design learning tasks within the complexity of the clinical setting. If students are to learn to think then the clinical teacher needs to determine what 'thought patterns' are required by the registered nurse. Learning strategies which enable students to practise those thought patterns as learners will provide preparation for professional practice as graduates. When the variety of clinical settings is considered, designing learning strategies to reflect specific thought patterns for practice requires considerable sophistication on the part of the clinical teacher. Stevens (1979) reminds us that, for the clinical teacher, teaching a functional role (as distinct from teaching content) involves the teacher in actually 'being as well as knowing'. In elaborating further, Stevens explains '(I)n role education, one not merely adds to the fund of knowledge of the student but also impacts on her (*sic*) very being. The roles that one fills in life become part of the self. Thus the educator in functional areas not only informs students but she (*sic*) forms them, and that is a more weighty responsibility' (p. 173).

There is yet another role for the clinical teacher which is perhaps more relevant to specialized settings than to the generalist settings where most undergraduate students are taught. Benner (1989) describes a role for the clinical teacher in 'making visible the expert knowledge in intensive care nursing' (p. 3). Later in her discourse, Benner asserts '(I)f we do not do a good job of teaching the human side and the caring practice side, then our graduates will not be in a good position to be safe and human clinical learners and practitioners. We dare not hold up a model of technical proficiency without equal proficiency and understanding of our caring practices' (p. 16).

The dual roles of teacher and carer spawn many debates. Where do the responsibilities of teacher and carer overlap, where should they be separate? Such debates usually hinge on the answer to questions such as: What are the primary responsibilities of the clinical teacher during a clinical teaching session? To whom is the clinical teacher responsible?

The conflict arising out of dual roles was recognized in the work of the Career Structure Committee of the Royal Australian Nursing Federation. The traditional structure in which there was no clear role for the clinical nurse and the clinical nurse consultant in teaching, and the nurse educator's role was mainly enacted in the classroom, has been replaced by a new structure which gives clinical nurses a clear career pathway and the nurse educator a teaching role in both classroom and clinical setting. Silver (1989) defines the nurse educator:

> The Nurse Educator's . . . responsibilities include teaching and clinical teaching activities for a specified group of students, staff and clinical units. He or she may co-ordinate a course or programme within the School of Nursing (p. 232).

Clearly, the responsibilities are for students, not patients. On the other hand, the Clinical Nurse Consultant is defined as

> an expert clinician who provides leadership and co-ordination of one clinical unit/service delivery team over which the incumbent has total authority. The role incumbent gives direct patient care to a small number of patients/clients with complex care needs on a regular basis in order to demonstrate his or her expertise. The incumbent acts as a process and expert consultant to the staff of the ward/unit, and as an expert consultant to other areas on request, in relation to his or her area of expertise (p. 232).

In these circumstances, the role of the clinical teacher is clear in that it is specified in relation to particular students, staff and clinical units. As it is unlikely that a clinical teacher would be 'expert' in all clinical settings or fields, the delineation of a specified clinical unit enables clinical teachers to keep abreast of developments in their clinical specialty field and to make sure that they continue to perform proficiently, as a teacher, in that clinical area.

Students look for both these roles in their teachers (Windsor, 1987). The clinical acumen of the teacher is important, as that knowledge and experience is used to assist students to synthesize theoretical concepts with practical realities and to provide opportunities for students to learn how the clinician thinks in action. The role of teacher as instructor rather than clinician is, however, also important and one in which many teachers feel the need to develop explicit skill.

The component skills of the instructor role have been defined in relation to supervisors in teacher education (Turney *et al.*, 1982, p. 85). The skills are defined as Presenting, Questioning, Problem Solving and Conferencing and each skill has several components:

1. *Presenting* has components of Suggesting, Modelling and Explaining.
2. *Questioning* has the following components: Lifting the level, Pausing, Probing, Asking divergent questions.
3. *Problem solving* has components of Delineating the problem, Identifying factors and gathering information, Seeking solutions, Applying and appraising solutions.
4. *Conferencing* has components of Planning for the conference, Guiding discussion and Terminating the conference.

There are some obvious similarities between these supervisory skills in teacher education and the instructor role in nurse education. While the term clinical teaching is preferred to the concept of supervision in nurse education, the same skills are exercised in the laboratory and pre- and post-conference sessions.

Kermode (1985) examined the concept of clinical supervision in teacher education and concluded that there is a similarity between the skills required for the supervision of a learner-teacher in the classroom and those for a clinical teacher in nursing, in a clinical setting. A critical difference, however, is that the supervisor is only an observer of the student-teacher, not an active partner in the lesson. In contrast the clinical teacher in nurse education has several options for participation. The teacher may take a purely supervisory role when that is appropriate for the level of student learning, the condition of the patient/client or the context, alternatively, the clinical teacher may act as observer, noting aspects of the performance for later discussion; but more usually, the clinical teacher is involved in the practice, by role modelling, instructing, assisting in the care by lifting or adjusting equipment or talking with the patient/client. At times immediate feedback may be necessary and the teacher may intervene to protect the patient/client and the student from a potentially hazardous or undesirable procedure.

It is helpful, therefore to think of a clinical learning triad of student, patient/client and teacher which requires skills beyond those which comprise the supervisory role in teacher-education.

According to Little and Ryan (1988) the instructor role in nurse education has become almost devoid of the traditional instructor skills of lecturing or presenting information, and in their place the role of facilitator of the students' self-directed learning has been adopted. The 'facilitator role demands an ability to help students to develop skills in critical thinking and problem-solving/reasoning, self-directed learning and self-evaluation' (p. 2). The teacher exercises this ability using strategies which constantly challenge the students' assumptions, understanding, knowledge base, and self-directed learning skills. Just as importantly, the teacher challenges the students' ability 'to identify their learning needs and ability to assess accurately their own performance' (p. 3).

Questioning skills are obviously basic to the facilitator's role. The questions, however, should not be the kind which ask for information or the 'right answer', but those which challenge the students to trace their own thinking strategies and to explain how they drew inferences or came to a certain conclusion.

The extent to which the instructor or facilitator roles are played depends on the philosophy of clinical teaching, the level of the students, and on the structure or system of clinical teaching adopted by a school or faculty. For example, if teachers espouse the principles of experiential learning (see Chapter 2) then the teacher will be predominantly a facilitator as the students will be encouraged to reflect on their experience and to draw insights from its meaning for them, and guidance for their future practice. If, on the other hand, clinical teaching is structured to include laboratory, pre-clinical and post-clinical sessions, as well as instruction during clinical practice, there will be a judicious mix of instructor and facilitator roles. Research for the clinical microskills teaching project (White *et al.*, 1988(a)) revealed that the skills exercised by clinical teachers during the clinical practice session were concerned mainly with giving informed support and guidance, implementing roles negotiated prior to the session, affirming judgements, and corrective intervention. The preparation undertaken in laboratory and pre-clinical sessions provided the students with sufficient confidence and skill to enable the clinical teacher to dispense with a 'supervisory/teaching' role during clinical practice and to use the post-conference session to follow up with the students their own assessment of their practice and of their learning.

The assessment of students' clinical performance places on clinical teachers not only a conflict of roles, but a need to be aware of the criteria for effective practice. In turn, this makes clinical teachers vulnerable in the light of their own standards of practice; their cherished practices may no longer be acceptable to the new policies and practices of performance. Students who regard their teacher as a role model might therefore perform in ways that meet her/his approval, but which may not meet the requirements of assessment in that school.

There is also a broader professional role for clinical teachers. Davis (1988) points to the importance of keeping in touch with new research in the areas of educational psychology and cognitive science. Developing knowledge in cognition, learning, memory and motivation signals the need for teachers to evaluate new research and to pilot new teaching/learning strategies.

The role of the clinical teacher in curriculum development also deserves mention. Integration of theory and practice is enhanced by curricula which present the theoretical component of the course as a preparation for clinical practice as well as a foundation for the discipline. The clinical teacher's role in curriculum evaluation should be an active one monitoring the extent to which the curriculum keeps pace with changes in the learners' needs. The role also involves contributing to curriculum content through clinical nursing research.

Assistance for clinical teachers

Although there is growing awareness of the complexities of clinical teaching, and of the needs of clinical students, little is available to assist teachers to improve their clinical teaching skills. Until recently, texts have been few and mostly theoretical and philosophical. New teachers in particular need a 'what to do, how to do guide', backed up by educational principles. Clinical teachers also need some knowledge of curriculum structure so that they can appreciate, understand and reinforce the major emphasis (for example, problem solving, concepts, competencies) in operation in the classroom.

The reality of pressures on today's health care system and its changing patterns demands teachers who can teach in both institutional and community care settings and who can assist the student's involvement in discharge planning and in the transition of patients from hospital to home. Assistance for clinical teachers to maintain their professional practice competencies is essential. This may take the form of clinical projects, release time for clinical refreshment, or such measures as joint appointments between clinical settings and educational institutions.

1.4 CHALLENGES

In addition to the challenge of the many roles of the clinical teacher, the changes in the health care and educational systems bring their own special demands.

Changes in the health care system

Mention has already been made of the early discharge of patients from hospital, the extra demand on domiciliary care and the need for clinical teachers to be able to teach in any setting, institutional and non-institutional. The closure of many hospital beds and the extended waiting time for clients for elective surgery opens new areas of clinical teaching in ambulatory and out patients' clinics and follow up care in the patients' homes. Students who are inexperienced in both life events and health/illness deviations require clinical teachers who can provide the necessary guidance, nursing skill and emotional support.

Short stay hospital admissions, the demands of short term surgical treatments, the changes to hospital administrative routines as a result of economic constraints, the pressures on staff and the consequent lower job satisfaction, have all influenced the environment for clinical teaching. Flexibility in teaching patterns is essential; clinical teaching cannot always be implemented as planned. More 'opportunistic' teaching is required; the clinical teacher must teach in unplanned sessions, using opportunities as they arise. This unpredictability can be alarming for many new clinical teachers whose prior teaching experience has been in the safety of the classroom and whose teaching practice has been based on objectives and carefully chosen strategies. It can also be turned to positive advantage since graduates must also master the skill of functioning within uncertainty. The clinical teacher's response to altered and unpredictable circumstances can be a positive model.

The principles of primary health care with its emphasis on the World Health Organization's theme 'Health for All' have been included in the majority of nursing curricula. Some curricula are built on primary health care as the fundamental framework. Clinical teachers need to take on board the skills of working not solely on a one-to-one basis, but as part of a primary health care team, guiding students to the differences between the concepts of nursing in primary health care and nursing in the system of primary nursing (Dowling *et al.*, 1982).

Changes in the educational system

More changes have occurred in the education of nurses in Australia, in the last decade, and have occurred more rapidly, than at any other time in the nation's history.

In a short span of years, after a long period of petitions for change from the nursing profession, nursing education moved out of hospital schools into the mainstream of general tertiary education. Hard upon that change, came another. This time, the higher education system itself was in the midst of change. With the aim of ending the binary system of higher education in Australia, the unified system provided a mechanism for Colleges of Advanced Education (CAEs) where most nursing education was located to be amalgamated with universities. Nurse education has therefore travelled from a hospital based apprenticeship system to a university based education in less than a decade.

What implications are there for the clinical teacher?

For clinical teachers the change from a hospital programme to a university programme has not only been the change from one institution to another, but from one organization in the health system, to an entirely different organizational structure in the education system. Becoming a member of the university faculty brought different challenges. For individual faculty the demands of scholarship, writing and research as well as teaching, maintaining clinical and professional credibility called for reserves of intellectual vitality and personal tenacity previously untested. Finding themselves with professional qualifications (the requirement for clinical practice and clinical teaching) but without parallel academic qualifications, teachers in nursing were at a disadvantage compared with their academic colleagues in other fields. Achieving higher educational qualifications has become essential.

What are the implications for clinical teaching?

Clinical teaching occurs within a very different framework from classroom teaching and it is true to say that the academic rigour of clinical teaching is at least as demanding. However, the recognition of the clinical programme as an academic endeavour with equivalent value in academic credit has been slow. There is continuing pressure to justify the depth of intellectual content of clinical practice in relation to the breadth, variety and brevity of its practice. The academic value of the clinical programme rests in the expertise necessary to manipulate the variables in clinical practice to make an educative environment; the skills of applying theoretical material to clinical practice; of integrating knowledge of biological, physical and social science perspectives appropriate for individual client's problems; of being able to select strategies for dealing with a student's learning problems as well as those appropriate for the application of specific theoretical concepts to individual client problems. Preparing students to make the kinds of judgements that will be part of their everyday professional activities cannot be said to be any less complex or cognitively demanding than the preparation of their colleagues in other professional fields.

What are the implications for clinical learners?

Students are often overwhelmed by their feelings when faced with the emotional impact of clinical nursing. Although the academic environment of the institution helps in analysing and talking through emotional difficulties and in preparing students for clinical experience, classroom or laboratory sessions cannot take the place of actual experience in the real setting. Certainly, explicit preparation for the unknown and unfamiliar is an improvement over the former traditional programmes where admission of one's fears to a teacher was unthinkable. Modern students rely on the relationship they have with their teachers and look to them to anticipate their difficulties, to encourage them and to give support, individually and personally.

The impact of higher education on learners has been studied extensively, from pressures of assignments and examinations, to class numbers and lecture hours load, and availability of textbooks and library access. For clinical students, the demands are considerable. Extra hours in clinical sessions, writing up of client studies and care plans, as well as travel to and from the clinical and educational institution add many hours to the weekly schedule. Students in tertiary nursing courses are now more demanding of their clinical teachers. With the expansion of the theoretical components of the course, they seek assistance in understanding complex concepts and in integrating knowledge from a number of subject areas before they are confident to use that knowledge in practice. The stimulation of the academic environment for learners and teachers has given clinical learners a new visibility.

Shared personal involvement in caring in clinical practice provides teachers and students with the additional experience of depth in interpersonal relationships. Sharing with teachers an increasing understanding of how nursing is practised is one of the more exciting opportunities for clinical learners in the 1990s.

What are the implications for clinical learning?

The conceptualization of clinical learning has evolved significantly since Nightingale's St Thomas' Hospital School of Nursing of the last century. Twentieth century theories of learning and instruction (Dewey, 1938; Ausubel, 1963; Bruner, 1966; Rogers, 1983; Gagne, 1976; Kolb, 1984; Schon, 1988) have drawn attention to the processes of learning and to the conditions necessary for learning to occur. Theories of nursing have stimulated a reconsideration of what it is that students are required to learn as clinical students (Fawcett, 1989).

The opportunity to plan clinical learning in an academic environment enabled clinical educators to review not only what and how students learn, but importantly, the organization of activities which facilitate clinical learning. The selection of learning experiences to accompany and exemplify the underlying theoretical foundations studied in the classroom has changed the nature of learning in clinical settings. Clinical assignments are more likely to be planned and defined in terms of the learning to be accomplished rather than sets of tasks to be completed.

Systems or models of clinical learning have been developed to meet the special demands of educating a variety of practising professionals. Schon's (1988) model of 'Educating the Reflective Practitioner' has raised questions about current professional training. According to Schon learners respond to coaching where the emphasis is on the student in relation to goals for learning rather than teaching for professional practice, where the emphasis is on the content or the teacher.

In nursing, Infante (1985) notes the emphasis on clinical learning in the conceptual frameworks of an increasing number of curricula and stresses the importance of the consistent use of a conceptual framework throughout all steps in the teaching/learning process. For example, if a particular nursing theory is selected as the conceptual framework then the concepts comprising the theory should permeate the students' learning and practice. Infante includes a proposed sequence of teaching/learning activities from classroom activities to clinical practice as a 'planned progression of teaching/learning activities' (p. 78) which supports the use of a chosen conceptual framework.

The approach to clinical learning proposed in the present text adopts a cyclical model (Figure 1.1) and is based on observations made in a number of nursing programmes in Australia (White *et al.*, 1988(a)). The progression of learning we observed began with the theoretical component of the programme, proceeded to a laboratory where principles and concepts from the theoretical component were applied and practised, then progressed to a briefing or pre-conference before clinical practice, followed by a debriefing or post-conference component. A further component was added in some programmes consisting of a follow-up session with students and all teachers, including basic science and central discipline teachers, to provide feedback and to provide the link between clinical learning and the programme as a whole. The model is similar to one which is based on research and used widely in teacher education (Goldhammer, 1969; Turney *et al.*, 1982; Smyth, 1986). Although undergoing continual refinement it has retained the important components of observation, pre-conference (briefing) and post-conference (debriefing).

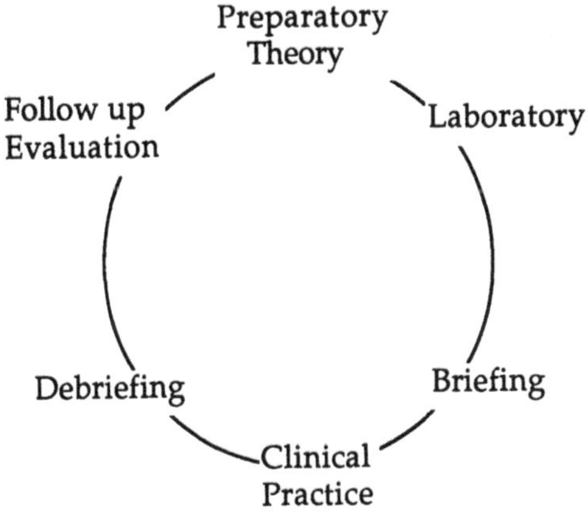

Figure 1.1 Clinical learning cycle.

Changes in the higher education system in Australia have influenced clinical learning. It is now a fruitful field for research and scholarship as well as for improved clinical practice. Until sufficient research is undertaken to reveal the nature of the learning task for students, the complexity of the environment in which learning takes place and the teaching skills required to facilitate students' understanding and professional development, the intellectual rigour of clinical learning and teaching will remain under-valued.

What are the implications for the patient/client?

Throughout this text the emphasis is on facilitating student learning through a variety of clinical teaching and learning strategies. At the outset the questions must be posed, 'What is the purpose? Who should benefit most from advances in learning and practice?' Certainly, students are learning a professional craft; teachers are improving their knowledge and skills. Ultimately, however, the improved care and future health of the consumer, client or patient must be the primary aim of the endeavour.

Students in modern nursing education programmes have many more options in providing care to clients. Initial learning, practising and being assessed in simulated settings protects patients from novices 'practising' for the first time. The presence of a clinical teacher or a mentor increases the possibility that standards of care will be maintained and a stronger emphasis on prevention in many programmes encourages an approach which informs patients about their illness and how to avoid complications.

1.5 FRAMEWORK OF THE BOOK

The clinical learning cycle provides the framework for the book. Chapter 1 has provided an overview of the nature of clinical teaching, its context and challenges. Key concepts and principles underlying many approaches to clinical teaching are discussed in Chapter 2. Chapter 3 begins consideration of the clinical learning cycle in the college laboratory. Teaching and learning alternatives are presented in a self-instructional style as in the remaining chapters. The briefing or pre-conference segment is the focus of Chapter 4; teaching and learning in clinical and community practice is the subject of Chapter 5, while Chapter 6 deals with debriefing and post-conference. The final chapter addresses the socialization process in becoming a nurse.

2

Foundations of clinical teaching and learning

2.1 INTRODUCTION

Effective clinical learning is a major objective in preparing professional nurses for the health care services. In the past, the constraints of hospital based schools and the demands of service on students' learning time have prevented a full realization of those aims.

The shift of nursing education into tertiary institutions provides new opportunities for planned clinical programmes and new challenges for teachers and researchers.

Given the importance of clinical teaching and learning in nursing, a dependable basis on which to plan and build effective teaching and learning practices is essential. Qualifications in education have long been expected of nurse educators, and short courses and inservice programmes have permitted updating of knowledge and skills. Without doubt, classroom teaching has benefited. Unfortunately, the relevance of educational theories to clinical teaching has not always been identified with equal enthusiasm. Given the challenges clinical teachers face and the complex environment in which clinical students learn, can an effective foundation for the practice of clinical teaching be found in educational theories? If so, which ones?

Obviously, clinical teaching is vastly different from teaching a discipline such as, for example, anatomy and physiology, pharmacology or microbiology. The aim of clinical teaching is to reinforce material already learned rather than to introduce new material. Unfortunately, many teachers have a preference for certain subjects and especially if they have a reputation for knowledge in an area, they will find opportunities to expound at the bedside. Clarification of the purpose of clinical teaching is long overdue. Both students and teachers suffer from confusion as to why they are in a particular clinical area and what they are supposed to learn, as distinct from what they are to do.

It is important to be clear that clinical teaching is not the same as teaching 'clinical' subjects, such as medical or surgical or paediatric nursing. Those subjects are studied within a theoretical framework whereby the student masters a defined set of knowledge as part of a formal programme or segment of curriculum. If this seems too fine a line to draw we should reconsider the definition offered in Chapter 1. In this text clinical teaching is defined as that which *prepares students to integrate their previously acquired knowledge with skills and competencies*. As students translate theory into practice, personal and professional skills, attitudes and behaviours are learned and practised in the care of clients or patients.

2.2 EDUCATIONAL FOUNDATIONS

In a survey of priorities in nursing education research (Tanner and Lindeman, 1987) six of the top ten research priorities related to clinical teaching. They are:

> What method of instruction best develops clinical problem-solving skills at baccalaureate and master's levels?
>
> What is the most effective approach to teaching clinical nursing skills?
>
> What clinical teaching strategies are more conducive to the development of professional qualities, e.g., critical thinking, accountability, change agent?
>
> What types of clinical performance evaluation strategies are most reliable and valid?
>
> What factors enhance the transfer of didactic learning into clinical practice? (Lindeman, 1989(a))

Most clinical teachers would agree that there are no surprises here since few research studies have addressed the problems at the heart of the questions. Several of the questions are of particular relevance to the educational foundations of curriculum construction and instructional design which, in turn, influence clinical teaching. The principles of learning upon which problem-based, concept-based and competency-based curricula are founded influence the design of clinical teaching. Clinical teaching draws upon many educational approaches; experiential learning, adult education, cognitive, behaviourist, developmental and humanistic theories.

Identification of the most effective approach or approaches to teaching clinical nursing skills is paramount. Time spent in laboratory teaching and in supervised clinical/community teaching is raised in the context of rising costs of education and limited access to clinical facilities. Other issues are equally demanding of resolution, such as: the workable balance between the emphasis on learning principles and the time actually spent in practising technical skills; bridging the gap between the skills practised in the lab and those required in the clinical setting; the comparative value of learning skills in the context of a clinical problem or mastering technical skills for application to many situations.

What assistance can be gained from educational theorists?

Ideally, a clinical learning theory would include elements of behaviourist, cognitive, humanistic and developmental learning theories. Many theorists have been considered in the search for an appropriate constellation for clinical learning. Duffy (1986) reviewed major theories of learning of the behaviourist and cognitive schools and concluded that conditioning theories, confined mainly to the learning of skills, have a limited place in nurse education. Certainly, the Skinnerian process of isolating the steps in performance to gain results on each element goes against the notion of 'holism' in learning skills. However, the behaviourist view of shaping behaviour with rewards can be useful in teaching psychomotor skills when the rewards for performance are given in terms of constructive feedback.

Duffy's (1986) comprehensive review leans towards cognitive learning theories because they can help to develop problem-solving skills, but recommends 'an eclectic approach to the application of the psychology of learning to daily teaching practice' (p. 26).

Russell (1980) also reviewed learning theories and conceptual models for clinical nursing, and drew upon Gagne's (1976) Learning Hierarchy as a model for teaching nursing skills.

The domains identified by Gagne: motor skills, verbal information, intellectual skills, cognitive strategies and attitudes point to different types of learning and provide a useful approach to planning clinical learning experiences. Bendall's (1977) proposition (cited by Russell, 1980, p. 42) that Gagne's theory is appropriate for teaching clinical nursing is explained in these terms:

> It means that the learner starts in reality, discovers and discriminates, is helped to categorise, and in discussion with a teacher builds categories into rules or principles, with the teacher feeding in extra essential knowledge at this stage.

This approach calls for well-developed skills in asking questions which require students to develop ability in discrimination, analysis, synthesis and evaluation.

Whilst Bloom's taxonomy of cognitive skills and Krathwohl's taxonomy of affective skills are useful in framing searching questions, there is an urgent need for a taxonomy of clinical learning skills. Such a taxonomy would combine the domains of cognitive, affective and psychomotor skills and provide for clinical application where all domains are acting at the same time. The interweaving of interpersonal skills with physical care which is so fundamental to nursing loses its richness when the two are treated as separate activities during the learning process.

Ausubel's cognitive theory is referred to in the paragraphs on concept learning (p. 26) below, and the work of theorists such as Dewey and Schon are included in the discussion on experiential learning (p. 30) which follows.

Most of the priority research questions identified in Tanner and Lindeman's (1987) study are framed in terms of *cognitive* skills. Humanistic theorists (Maslow 1954; Rogers 1969; Knowles, 1975), however, proclaim the need for involving feelings as well as intellect in learning. The self-enhancing process of such learning results in students becoming mature adults with openness to change and the skill to self-evaluate.

Roger's use of small groups where the teacher is friend and guide provide a model for briefing and debriefing sessions in clinical learning. Maslow's emphasis on self-enhancement provides an insight into motivation where learners see the possibility of achieving personal goals as well as fulfilling the requirements of the program. Knowles' (1975) well known approach to contract learning depends on the learners' concept of themselves as independent learners, able to decide what it is they want to learn, how to learn it, and how to achieve optimum results. Contract learning has gained a place in clinical learning (Bouchard and Steels, 1980; Sasmor, 1984; Gibbon, 1989).

Reilly and Oermann (1985) present a conceptual framework for teaching and learning 'derived from cognitive field theory and the ideas of others who perceive learning from a human science point of view' (p. 38). Cognitive field theory with its stress on problem solving and decision making is applicable to clinical learning.

> The role of perception, insight, meanings, relationships, and principles in learning and the transfer of learning is the essence of learning.Dewey's theory of experiential learning provides criteria for determining the educational value of the clinical experience. Bruner's stress on the importance of teaching the structure of knowledge (its meaningfulness and its relatedness) suggests the approach to teaching nursing's body of knowledge; Carl Roger's concern about the role of education in moving people toward self-actualization provides the stimulus to support the growth and development of the person who is to be the nurse. Perry's thesis about the need for education to move individuals from dualistic thinking to relativistic thinking and commitment challenges nursing teachers to enable students to deal with the uncertainties of a field which is an inexact science. Witkin's work on the significance of cognitive style in learning behaviour provides another basis for understanding learner needs and responses in the clinical practice site while Hall's and Mead's theses about cultural influences on the learning process provide new insight into a dimension of learning which has had little emphasis heretofore (Reilly and Oermann, 1985, p. 38).

The educational foundations for nursing curricula are based like Reilly and Oermann (1985) on a variety of theories, into which ideological, educational and professional nursing approaches can be accommodated. Some of the principal approaches and frameworks are discussed below.

Problem-based learning

It is not surprising to find that problem-based learning has become popular in health professions' education. What is surprising is that it has taken so long for it to be accepted. The work of Dewey, early this century, suggested that problem-solving was a legitimate form of human inquiry and that organizing the work of students around significant problems was the best way to encourage critical intelligence, and led to a break with traditional curricular patterns (Mason, 1972). Problem-solving is, of course, a characteristic feature of the activities of many professionals but the introduction of problem-based learning in the health professions was slow to develop. The medical programme at McMaster University, Canada, became entirely problem-based in the early 1970s, and several other medical programmes followed, for example Maastricht in The Netherlands and Newcastle, Australia. In the mid-1980s the nursing program at Macarthur Institute of Education (now the University of Western Sydney, Macarthur) introduced a problem-based course. Problem-based nursing curricula are organized around a contiguous learning framework, from clinical problems derived from practice and brought to the classroom, to clinical practice in a health care setting. Integration of content around problems identified as relevant, important and characteristic of professional practice forms the curriculum strategy. The problem-based curriculum gives the student practice in the classroom in selecting the content required from a number of sources (for example, formal subjects, resource persons, libraries and laboratories) for application to hypothetical clinical problems. Problem-solving skills are acquired during the process. The purpose of clinical teaching in such a programme is to assist the students to identify the client's problem, the knowledge to understand and resolve the problem and the skills they need to provide the client's care.

The student learns how to integrate theoretical material appropriately in relation to a variety of clinical problems which is an excellent preparation for clinical practice. For the clinical teacher, the model provides guidelines for planning the clinical learning cycle, the laboratory, briefing and debriefing sessions as well as the clinical practice session.

The decision to use the problem-based learning method in the Macarthur College Diploma of Applied Science (Nursing) programme was based on the belief that this method could best reflect the activities of nursing practice. Simulated problem situations could involve students in integrating their knowledge and applying it to clinical judgements, often in situations which are changing and complex. The necessity to use research and analytical skills in the problem-based method of learning provides students with a basis for future professional skills. Situation Improvement Packages (SIPs) devised by the faculty are based on actual clinical cases which place the students with patients in typical clinical situations. Students are required to respond to the situations and must plan appropriate care. The package incorporates a series of changed situations which mirror the patient's progress and the students are provided with a sequence of resources as the problem develops and as the students indicate a need for more information. 'Learning issues arise out of the exploration of the package, and the student pursues these using a variety of resources' (Ryan, 1989). Examples of the use of SIPs are given in Chapter 3.

Problem-based learning requires special teaching skills. An overly directive teacher can restrict the students' freedom to reason and prevent them from learning on their own. The tutor must guide, not direct; facilitate learning, not dispense information; keep interactions between students alive and the problem-based learning process on the track. The tutor must be certain that each student contributes and that the process is active and stimulating. The tutor must give the students every opportunity to learn by discovery. The tutor must be able to establish a climate of openness that allows the students to say what they believe or know without fear of censure or ridicule. Learning can only occur when beliefs and ideas can be freely expressed (Barrows, 1984).

In turn, the students change from passive receivers of information to active controllers of their learning. In discussing the adjustment that students must make Ryan (1989) notes that some negative reactions can be anticipated from students expecting a more traditional information-receiving approach. The issue of appropriate faculty development is important as the role of guide or facilitator is not usually within the experience of many faculty members. Some teachers may have problems as they interpret the critical questions of students as a threat to their authority. Students who express their opinions openly, often in disagreement with the teacher, may be regarded as disrespectful and rebellious. Students' learning problems become more visible in problem-based courses, whereas in traditional didactic courses such problems are usually unnoticed. The extra time and skill involved in assisting students may be resented by teachers.

> Learning to teach in a problem-based manner, as with any other skill, therefore, requires intellectual change, will take extra time, and will be resisted, in a system which provides no academic recognition for educational sophistication (Thompson and Williams, 1985, p. 202).

What are the implications for the clinical teacher of the problem-based method of learning? How does the clinical teacher guide the student in making the step from the problem-based packages in the tutorial, to the actual situation and the real patient in clinical practice?

Concept learning

Other educators, while acknowledging that problem-solving is a necessary nursing skill, have chosen not to use a problem-based curriculum model. Instead, they have drawn on educational theorists such as Ausubel (1963) and Novak (1977) who formulated the notion of concept learning as a basis for curriculum integration and clinical teaching. Such curricula integrate theoretical material on the basis of concepts rather than problems. The central idea of such curricula is Ausubel's (1963) theory of meaningful learning. According to this theory, meaningful learning is the process by which new information is related to relevant existing information in an individual's knowledge structure. Ausubel refers to 'subsuming concepts' as the point of assimilation for new knowledge. New meaningful learning results in changes to an existing concept, which is modified or broadened according to the nature of the new knowledge (Novak, 1977). When an individual does not already possess basic relevant concepts rote learning, not meaningful learning, occurs. An example would be a new subject area which bears no relation to anything in the individual's experience. When the individual is familiar with the new material and is able to recognize relationships with existing information, relevant concepts 'subsume' the new information.

The attractiveness of this model is that content can be integrated according to major and minor concepts. Subject headings take their title from the major concept of the area which very often reflects a phenomenon relevant to nursing rather than the traditional subject nomenclature. Each subject's major and minor concepts act as core centres for learning and practice. These are carried over into clinical practice so that the students learn to recognize and integrate relevant concepts into their practice across a variety of conditions and settings.

The questioning skills of the teacher are obviously important in assisting students to recognize concepts and to differentiate between them. Integrating new concepts by forming links between one concept and another can also be encouraged through questions which are aimed at stimulating students to evaluate and analyse information.

The notion of 'advance organizers' was first introduced by Ausubel in 1960 to provide a 'cognitive bridge' for the introduction of new knowledge. Later he stated that 'the principal function of the organizer is to bridge the gap between what the learner already knows and what he needs to know before he can successfully learn the task at hand' (Ausubel, 1960, p. 148, quoted in Novak, 1977,

p. 80). This has implications for instructional strategies since the facilitation of new learning depends upon the teacher's knowledge of what the student already knows. In other words each block of new learning depends for its successful mastery on the adequacy of the existing concepts (Novak, 1977). Retrieval of concepts and application of previous learning to clinical situations is easier because the links between existing knowledge and new clinical situations are already established in the preclinical phase.

How can this be done in nursing education and in clinical learning and teaching? What are the implications for the clinical teacher? How can the clinical teacher guide the student in moving from the conceptual approach in the theoretical course to the application of concepts to clinical practice?

Competency-based learning

Another mechanism that has been used in curriculum development to assist students to translate theory into practice is based on a set of competencies. These are complex performance descripters which include skills, attitudes and behaviours and imply a specific set of knowledge. The context in which the competencies will be practised is also specified. A clear and precise listing of the components of professional competence is essential as a basis for the design of the programme, the selection of content and the teaching and learning strategies. Clusters of competencies provide the guide to the selection and integration of content. The student learns to extract knowledge from the theoretical component of the program to meet the competency to be practised.

Changes in nurse education resulting from the introduction of nursing into colleges and universities have influenced the examining and accrediting role of the registering authorities. In place of a final state examination the registering authorities have moved toward statements of competencies to be achieved throughout the course.

Defining competencies, however, can be a complex activity. For, as McGaghie *et al.* (1978) point out, attempting to find a universal definition of competence for any health profession may be impracticable as professional practice depends not just on the tasks to be performed but on health care needs and resources, the structure of the health care system and political, social and economic circumstances.

Cameron (1989) describes the difficulties in attempts to develop competency statements for Australian nursing practice. The search for 'a statement of competencies which represent the total behavioural repertoire of the registered nurse (which) would do much to define the role of the nurse' (p. 210) is occupying the registering authorities. Such a statement would also pre-empt the introduction of a nursing practice act in Australia by defining the scope of nursing practice.

It is the broad nature of competencies which poses a problem for clinical teachers (Pratt, 1989). The determination of exactly which psychomotor skills the beginning practitioner needs to learn and master is impeded. '. . . it is the very global nature of the term (competencies) which has masked the specificity of subsumed skills and militated against their identification – an identification which would appear crucial in terms of preparing qualified practitioners who can demonstrate the requisite behavioural repertoire' (p. 20). Pratt's definition of a competency as depicted in Figure 2.1 below exemplifies the problem.

The problematic nature of the identification of nursing skills raised by the competencies issue demands a re-assessment of the value of task analysis and questions the accuracy of 'armchair' contemplation of practice. The issue of designing practice for future roles rather than present tasks inevitably surfaces. Cameron (1989) advocates the observation of practice as the way to derive competencies, and presumably the preferred method of identification of the skills necessary to achieve the competency.

According to Swendsen-Boss (1985) competencies 'derive from roles and emphasize performance rather than just knowledge', and

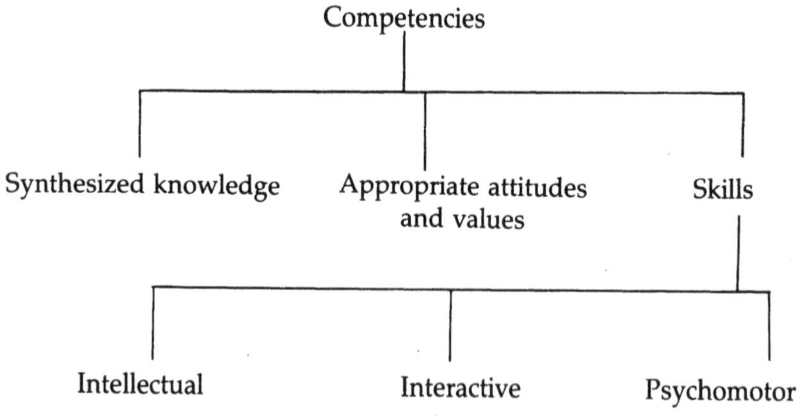

Figure 2.1 Definition of a competency.

Source: Pratt, (1989).

'clinical judgement not psychomotor skill' (p. 9). A clear statement of how competencies can be stated is helpful:

1. the conditions under which a student performs;
2. the actions or behaviours;
3. the standard of performance.

For example:

> Given a post op. client (condition), the student will assess fluid and electrolyte status and implement nursing intervention (action) that will assist the client to maintain fluid and electrolyte balance (standard) (p. 9).

The nature and organization of learning experiences in a competency-based programme are essentially those that enable mastery of the competencies. If the goal of the programme is to achieve professional competence, then progressive demonstration of that competence is a major feature of the student's progress through the course. What are the implications for the clinical teacher of a programme based on competencies? How can the clinical teacher assist students to demonstrate their use of the underlying knowledge appropriate to the performance of the competency?

Much has been written about the concept and practice of mastery learning (Block, 1971) which is relevant to competency-based curricula and need not be repeated here. What are the implications for clinical learning? The essential features of mastery learning are that competencies are introduced in sequential steps, first in the college laboratory where mastery can be demonstrated; then the competency is performed in the clinical setting. Some of the more complex competencies requiring administration of services, or community involvement, will obviously require a longer span of time for the performance to be assessed.

Generally, the mastery method requires that students gain immediate feedback on performance, both in the college laboratory and clinical settings. Self-pacing by the student is also a key concept and has a definite place in clinical learning. The implications for the clinical teacher are that time is required in planning the sequential steps, supporting and prompting students towards attainment of competencies, and in managing the roles of teacher and assessor. Encouraging students to assess their own attainment and their further learning, while important in any clinical teaching, is a skill that has direct implications for success of the mastery model and the sequence of further learning experiences.

While the curriculum may be designed primarily on a problem-based, concept-based or competency-based model, it may also draw on the principles of problem-solving, concept learning or competency attainment as appropriate to learning how to perform in professional practice.

Experiential learning

It is both interesting and instructive to read the works of John Dewey (1938) on experience and education. He describes the experiences offered in traditional education which were, largely, the wrong kind. How many students, he asks, 'were rendered callous to ideas, and how many lost the impetus to learn because of the way in which learning was experienced by them? How many acquired special skills by means of automatic drill so that their power of judgment and capacity to act intelligently in new situations was limited?' (p. 26). One could imagine he wrote especially about nurse education! His message is that it is not enough simply to include experiences in learning: everything depends on the quality of the experience. Planning experiences is important. It is important to provide continuity rather than separate and discrete experiences that have little possibility of providing an experiential continuum.

> . . . the central problem of an education based on experience is to select the kind of present experiences that live fruitfully and creatively in subsequent experiences (Dewey, 1938, p. 28).

How do students learn from experience?

Dewey foreshadowed the need for a theory of experience which would give direction to the selection and organization of appropriate educational methods and materials. One such theory has been proposed by Kolb (1984). Kolb's theory explains the process of experiential learning as having concrete experiences, reflective observation, abstract conceptualization and active experimentation. These processes have been adopted in some nursing programmes to provide a framework for clinical education.

Kolb's theory has formed the basis for study of the way experience can be transformed into knowledge. The Boud *et al.* (1985) model of experience-based learning sets out the reflective processes that can be used to assist students to gain meaning from their experiences (Figure 2.2).

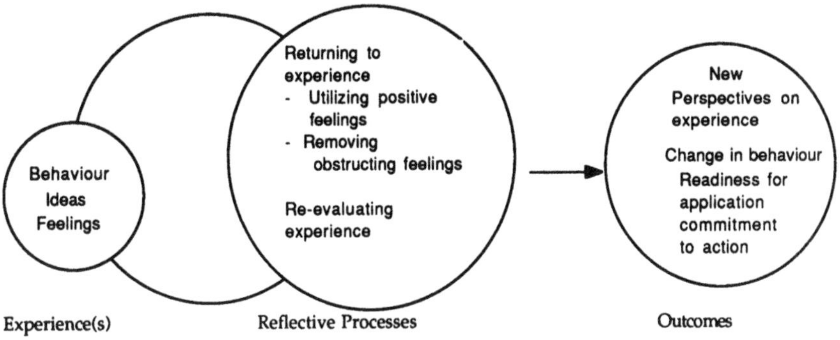

Figure 2.2 The reflection process.

Source: Boud (1988).

Since most field or clinical education programmes are designed around students' real experiences, it is self-evident that experiential learning theories and models are relevant to clinical education. For example Boud's model, used in the pre- and post-conferences in clinical teaching, provides a guide for clinical teachers.

Reflecting about experience enables its meaning to be grasped and its potential for future practice to be explored. Reflecting during practice 'reflection-in-action' (Schon, 1988) takes us into practice itself. In Schon's words,

> We may reflect on action, thinking back on what we have done in order to discover how our knowing-in-action may have contributed to an unexpected outcome. We may do so after the fact, in tranquility, or we may pause in the midst of action to make what Hannah Arendt (1971) calls a 'stop-and-think.' In either case, our reflection has no direct connection to present action. Alternatively we may reflect in the midst of action without interrupting it. In an action-present – a period of time, variable with the context, during which we can still make a difference to the situation at hand – our thinking serves to reshape what we are doing while we are doing it, I shall say in cases like this that we reflect-in-action (p. 26).

Schon (1988) uses the term 'professional artistry' in his book *Educating the Reflective Practitioner* to describe the competence of practitioners in 'unique, uncertain and conflicted situations of practice' (p. 22). The artistry he speaks of strikes a chord with nurses as they also recognize the components of artistry in their thinking and practice. Schon describes the tools of professional artistry in the following terms. We become skilful in the use of a tool as we learn to 'appreciate, directly and without intermediate reasoning, the qualities of the materials that we apprehend through the tacit sensations of the tool in our hand' (p. 23). While it is often impossible to describe the spontaneous recognitions we make, or how we make them, the ability to learn new skills is, in part, attributable to these tacit sensations. Schon gives examples, such as learning to ride a bicycle, without being able to describe how we do it. He calls this knowing-in-action; 'the knowing is in the action', (p. 25). 'Know*ing* suggests the dynamic quality of knowing-in-action, which, when we describe it, we convert to know*ledge*-in-action' (p. 26).

Readers who are familiar with the works of Benner (1982, 1984, 1989) will recognize similarities with her notion of skilled clinical knowledge. Clinical knowledge to Benner is knowledge which is embedded in the practice of nursing. Just as the connoisseur is able to make fine discriminations without being able to give a description of how a critical judgement is made, so expert nurse clinicians become connoisseurs of subtle patient changes (Benner and Wrubel, 1982a).

How might we approach clinical learning and teaching in order to encourage knowing-in-action and skilled clinical knowledge? Schon describes a method of teaching a new skill (learning to play tennis) as helping students to get the feel of 'hitting the ball right' and learning to distinguish those feelings from 'hitting the ball wrong'. Schon also describes how reflection enables exploration of any new observations we make and testing of new actions we may invent. Reflection-in-action has a questioning, critical component, urging us to challenge previous thinking and the assumptions underlying our knowing-in-action.

Benner talks of perceptual awareness and skilled clinical knowledge development. The 'aspects' of a nursing or client situation are recognized and acted upon only when we have enough prior experience and knowledge-in-action to be able to discriminate among relevant and unimportant cues or aspects. For Benner, the essential thing about reflection is that it is a reflection more on *practice*, than on *theory* (Benner, 1989). Clinical teachers play an essential role in helping students to reflect on their practice and in enlarging each student's understanding of its meaning.

Classroom teaching has through a firm educational foundation a long history of support, a variety of theorists and research which provides a base for new methods and strategies. Clinical teaching in the health professions must also depend on a sound educational foundation. Research to identify that foundation is long overdue.

2.3 NURSING THEORY FOUNDATIONS

What can be drawn from nursing theories which would provide a foundation for clinical teaching and learning? Theory development in nursing has both an exciting and a frustrating history. It is a history characterized by many adherents and not a few sceptics. To trace the literature on theoretical thinking in nursing from the 1960s is to gain a sense of urgency, industry, innovation and, some would say, pretension. Caught up in the whirl of ideas have been educators, administrators and practitioners who have been tantalized by the notions of a body of knowledge which distinguishes nursing as a discipline in its own right.

The early attempts to establish a theoretical basis for nursing have been traced by several authors (Newman, 1979; Riehl and Roy 1980; Kim 1983; Fawcett, 1983; Marriner, 1986). Other authors have provided texts detailing the structural components of their models and theories. An overview of conceptual models and theories is given in Fawcett (1989).

The emergence of theory has accompanied, both nationally and internationally, a concern which has been expressed in many ways, particularly in the late 1970s (Putt, 1978; Stevens, 1979). The concern is that, although nursing practice is complex and draws on a number of disciplines, yet, it is in danger of remaining a practice based on a repertoire of routines, rituals and habits until its theoretical directions are more clear.

The issue is alive and fosters interesting debates. Many nurses would agree with Benner that a nursing theory is yet to be developed which starts from practice as it is performed at the present time by expert nurse practitioners (Benner, 1989). They would also be in sympathy with Chinn and Jacobs (1983) who claim that 'most nursing theory represents the nursing world as it ought to be or might be, which is quite different from the nursing world in which practitioners function'. Nor is it surprising that the theorist and the practitioner might find themselves at odds, although there is no doubt that they need each other. While the theorist seeks principles and laws which are highly generalizable (and therefore abstract), the practitioner also seeks principles and laws which because of their level of generality can be transferred from one clinical situation to the next (Duhamel, 1982).

Taking the middle ground Storch (1986) seeks to allay the fears of sceptics in her paper 'In defence of nursing theory'. For those nurses to whom 'in the thick of nursing practice, nursing theory just seems like so many words when there's work to be done', Storch relates to the value of theory-directed nursing in increasing the level of knowledge and understanding for the benefit of enhanced patient care.

The crux of the issue for clinical teaching and learning is how should nursing theories be used as a basis for nursing practice? Is it necessary to base clinical teaching and learning on a particular nursing theory or model? Which nursing theories can we trust?

One of the hallmarks of a profession is said to be the framework for professional practice; to challenge the models or theories on which patterns of clinical practice have been built. With the expansion of nursing into tertiary education in Australia, the philosophical and theoretical base of its practice has been brought into open debate. Emden (1988) sought the opinions of nursing leaders in Australia by Delphi probe, in an attempt to generate discussion on issues surrounding theory development in nursing. Emden reports that leading Australian nurses recognize many pathways to nursing knowledge and that while most consider that models of nursing are 'critical' to the advancement of nursing, they also emphasize that their importance was related to their capacity to enable the 'nature of nursing to be examined in depth thus leading to a clearer definition of nursing' (Emden, 1988, p. 31).

What has been the result of the attempts to apply nursing theories to clinical nursing? Several Australian educators seeking models or theories to guide curriculum development in new courses have explored the concepts and challenged the feasibility of basing a course on a specific conceptual model or theory. Two studies are discussed below.

Kermode (1987) reports on a study of the nursing programme at the Riverina Murray Institute of Higher Education (RMIHE) (now the Charles Sturt University). Specifically, the study aimed to discover whether when implemented, 'a curriculum based on a conceptual framework results in students using the concepts which the framework describes in a way that indicates the concepts are of use to the students'. Using a modification of an activities of daily living model of Roper *et al.* (1983) and concepts from both Henderson (1966) and Roy (1970), the RMIHE construct of nursing practice was developed (Figure 2.3).

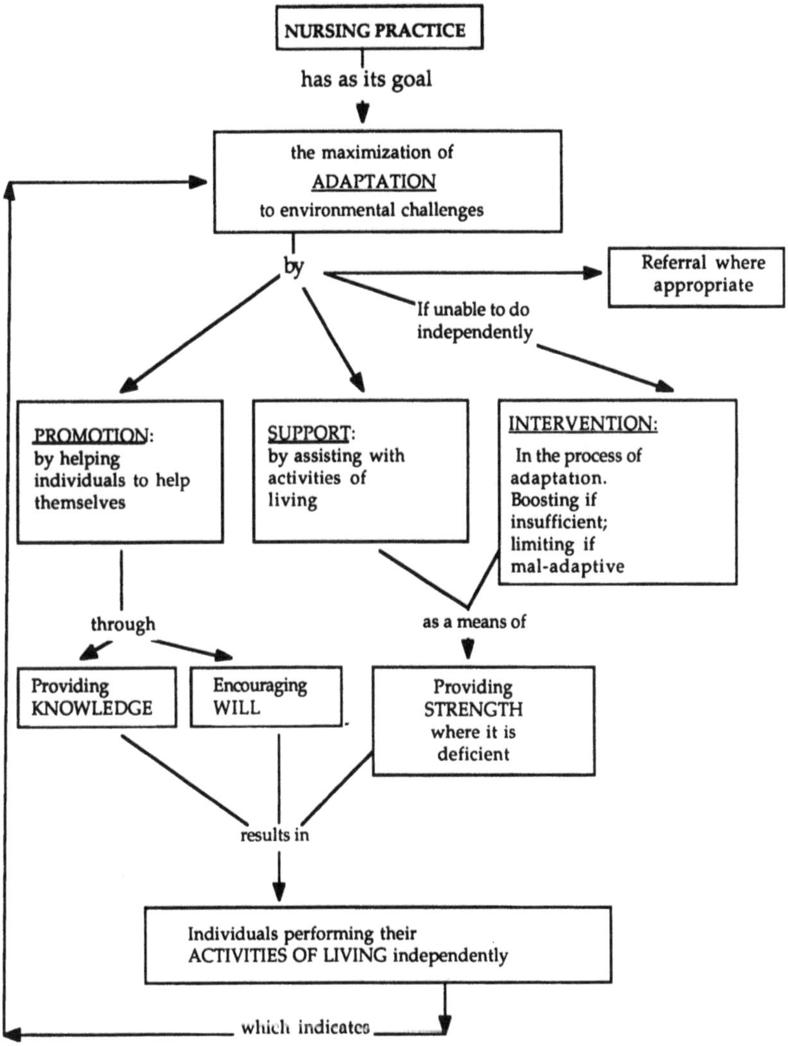

Figure 2.3 Construct of nursing practice.
Source: Kermode (1987).

Kermode tested students in their first year on their recognition, articulation and application of a group of concepts representative of the conceptual framework which have direct relationship to clinical practice. A problem-solving instrument was used, designed to examine how students think about patient problems, their causes and the appropriate nursing actions. A structured interview sought to gain additional information about the thinking behind students' judgements in the clinical setting. The aim was to determine which of the concepts in the conceptual framework of their programme were of use to them in their organization of their clinical practice and in dealing with real patient problems.

His results showed that students can, over time, improve significantly their ability to recognize and articulate a number of concepts on which the nursing curriculum is based. The results are not so positive in respect of the students' ability to apply the concepts in planning care for real patients, although they do give evidence of using concepts in deciding how to plan care in simulated situations.

Although the popularity of constructing and using a specific conceptual framework based on nursing models and theories has lost some of its support among nurse educators, the findings of this study are, nevertheless, important for clinical teaching. As we noted at the beginning of this chapter, the link between the theoretical programme and clinical learning provided by the curriculum structure is important in determining the students' success in integrating and applying content to clinical practice. It is reasonable to suggest that more advanced students than those in Kermode's study, with assistance in reflecting on the concepts they use in practice, could be expected to apply the concepts of their programme to their practice in a direct way. The study also reveals that the use of simulations based on a set of relevant concepts provide a valuable teaching tool and a method of self-assessment.

In another study conducted at the University of Wollongong, Partridge (1989) examined Orlando's (1961) claim that her 'disciplined professional response' typifies professional nursing practice. Partridge observed nursing activity in medical/surgical wards. The view taken in the study was that 'If Orlando has described what nursing is, as distinct from what it could or should be, then nursing activities should resemble, to a greater or lesser extent, the nursing process as she has defined it' (p. 95).

Partridge's results show that, 'Although some of the concepts which feature in the theory are seen as important by nurses they are not consistently part of nursing practice' (p. 114). Nevertheless, the results are instructive in respect of clinical teaching. The difference between Partridge's study and the study by Kermode is, of course, that Orlando's theory had not been used in the nursing programmes in which the subjects (registered nurses) had been students, and furthermore they had come from a variety of programmes. Whether their observed practice would have been different if they had been educated in a programme where Orlando's theory was the basis of the curriculum remains an open question.

Partridge concedes that 'there may be differences between those nurses who have completed hospital based courses and those who have completed tertiary courses in regard to their willingness to apply nursing theory to clinical practice. If tertiary study leads to a greater breadth and depth of understanding of the theoretical concepts of a discipline, then there should be a correlation between the level of the nurse's academic preparation and his/her sensitivity to the applicability of nursing theories' (p. 114).

An interesting issue is raised by Partridge. Claiming that the priority for future research lies in studies of the application of nursing theories to nursing practice, Partridge advocates research which would identify the nursing theories which can direct clinical care and their special areas of applicability. He recognizes that the multiplicity of theories impedes the task of identifying their special relevance to a variety of particular clinical nursing problems and leaves open the issue of whether the profession can or should attempt to identify specific theory–problem links.

What is the utility of nursing theories as a foundation for clinical teaching and learning? Considering that 'Nursing theories are under-investigated and have been developed for curriculum building rather than for or from practice' (Benner and Wrubel, 1989, p. 5, citing Meleis, 1985) the question challenges the nature of nursing itself. Benner and Wrubel (1989) claim that '[A] theory is needed that describes, interprets, and explains not an imagined ideal of nursing, but actual expert nursing as it is practiced today. This type of theory could be used to develop curricula in which practice informs nursing education in a way that nursing education has always influenced practice' (p. 5).

Must clinical teaching and learning wait for such a theory? The researchers in clinical teaching cited below have not waited and have begun where Benner claims theory should emerge, that is, in practice.

The nature of clinical teaching

What can be said about the study of the nature of clinical teaching itself? Two recent studies can be applied to the cycle of clinical learning, from theory, laboratory, pre- and post-conferences and clinical practice sessions. Chuaprapaisilp's (1989) study examines the changes necessary in teachers and students so that experiential learning can be planned and captured through pre- and post-clinical conferences. Carr's (1983) close observation of clinical teachers uncovers the dimensions of clinical teaching and delineates the components which could be applied to all stages of the clinical learning cycle.

Towards a model of critical experiential learning in clinical teaching?

When Chuaprapaisilp (1989) investigated pre- and post-clinical teaching in a nursing programme in Thailand, the aim was to find ways clinical teachers could use to improve their students' clinical learning. In what was a highly structured tradition of content-centred and teacher-centred programmes, the teachers, through workshop discussions, agreed that change was necessary. They produced an embryonic framework of experiential learning which was implemented during the study. As the action research progressed, the model changed several times to reflect better what teachers and students were learning about their experiences.

The model worked successfully to the extent that the teachers began to question not only the time-honoured way they had practised and taught in the past, but also the context, attitudes, cultures and sub-cultures that had made it so. This led to the surprising conclusion, in the Thai context, that their students also should learn to be critical within the supportive and emancipative framework of the experiential learning model. Chuaprapaisilp concluded that her study extended the reflective processes of the Boud *et al.* model (1988) see p. 31 above) to include 'gaining emancipation through experience' (Chuaprapaisilp, 1989, p. 254) and suggested questions to prompt students to discover other approaches to improve their experience, to learn to question the system, and to change attitudes. Gaining 'emancipation' through experience has relevance in clinical teaching and learning in both institutional and community settings.

Towards a theory of clinical teaching?

Carr (1983) conducted a study of clinical teachers who were full-time members of an undergraduate baccalaureate programme in a School of Nursing in Boston, USA. The teachers held responsibilities for both classroom and clinical teaching in medical–surgical nursing.

Descriptive data of clinical teaching derived from observation and from the teachers' point of view were obtained using symbolic interaction as the theoretical perspective. The results of the study offer a data base for developing a theory of clinical teaching in nursing grounded in practice. Carr's definition of clinical teaching which emerged from the investigation describes how the features she observed inter-relate. The definition offers 'a structure and a way of thinking about the realities of clinical teaching' (p. 339). Clinical teaching is

> a time limited process whereby the teacher and student create an established partnership within a shared environment in such a way that the teacher's primary, operational frame of reference is maintained as the legitimate means for affecting the student's behaviour toward intended purposes (Carr, 1984, p. 339).

Carr developed an information-processing model of clinical teaching which represents the elements in the definition. Through these elements (or educational realities) 'students are likely to learn certain knowledge, skills, qualities and values' (p. 340).

Carr's study is important in showing that it is possible to develop a structure descriptive of clinical teaching which could lead to a theory – not of clinical learning – but of clinical teaching. In raising the issue that 'theories of learning are inadequate as theories of teaching' (p. 385) Carr poses many questions about what it is that clinical teachers do to influence students' behaviour and learning.

What researchers such as Chuaprapaisilp and Carr have attempted for clinical teaching and learning mirrors what Benner intends for nursing practice and nursing care. 'Though nursing practice depends on science, nursing care requires more than science for its legitimacy and direction' (Benner, 1989, p. 20). Whilst clinical teaching and learning depends on educational psychology, the practice of teaching within the context of nursing care requires more than an educational foundation for its legitimacy and direction. The research included in Leininger and Watson (1990), *The Caring Imperative in Education*, indicates a move toward identifying within the complexities of caring those aspects students need to learn and the clinical teacher needs to foster in the clinical teaching triad of student, teacher and patient/client.

This chapter has given an overview of the key concepts and organizing principles underlying many approaches to clinical teaching and learning. Relevant theories in nursing and education have been presented and their utility for planning and conducting clinical teaching and assisting clinical learners has been discussed. The next three chapters will draw on some of this material as it relates to practical issues in each stage of the clinical learning cycle.

3

Learning in the laboratory

3.1 INTRODUCTION

Chapters 1 and 2 raised some of the important issues facing clinical teachers in nursing and explored the theoretical foundations upon which clinical learning and teaching may be based. Each of the following chapters draws on that material and relates it to the practice of clinical teaching. Using a self-instructional style a number of activities are suggested to enable you to draw on your own teaching practice as the basis for analysis and consideration of alternative approaches. Although the feedback which follows the activities can be read as a text in the usual way there are advantages in applying the practical examples provided to your own experience. The questions and activities may trigger ideas for your own teaching which may go unrecognized if the text is read without a gentle nudge from time to time.

3.2 THE CLINICAL LEARNING CYCLE

Each chapter in the remainder of the text takes a component of the clinical learning cycle as its focus (Figure 3.1). The purpose of the laboratory, briefing or preconference, the clinical practice session, and debriefing or post-conference are examined, and the design of the teaching and learning session, the possible teaching and learning processes and a variety of instructional strategies are included.

Strictly speaking, the clinical learning cycle begins with the major principles and concepts taught in the theoretical programme. For the purposes of this book, however, we are concerned only with teaching in those phases of the cycle which do not occur in the traditional

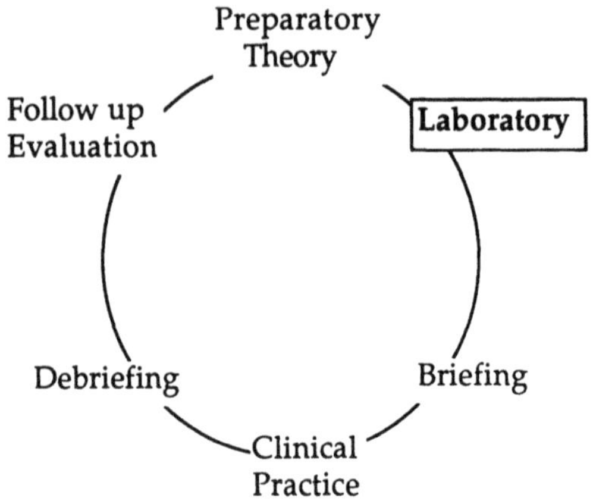

Figure 3.1 Clinical learning cycle: laboratory.

classroom setting. Clinical teachers may certainly use a variety of classroom teaching strategies in laboratories, briefing and debriefing sessions (for example, group work, role play, games and simulations and microskills such as reinforcement, explanation and questioning) and there are many general texts on teaching methods which deal with these skills specifically (for teaching skills relevant to teaching nursing see, for example, Ewan and White, 1984; de Tornyay, 1982).

The purpose of the chapter is to explore ways in which the laboratory can be used to assist students to understand and use concepts from the theoretical programme so that application to practice is achieved. By the end of this chapter you should be able to design a laboratory teaching session which is:

1. based on learning theories;
2. based on the model of nursing used by your school;
3. designed to develop students' intellectual and practical nursing skills.

Active debate characterizes discussions about what clinical skills students should learn (Kieffer, 1984; Field *et al.*, 1984; Aggleton *et al.*, 1987) and where, (Gomez and Gomez, 1987), when, how and how much they should learn (Elliott *et al.*, 1982; Sweeney *et al.*, 1982). Infante's (1985) approach is to emphasize the benefits of college laboratory activities and to suggest that 'preclinical conferences with a group of student tends to become unnecessary' (p. 85). On the other hand, Lindeman (1989(a)) suggests that clinical teaching must place less emphasis on 'pre-experience grill and drill' and more on inclusion of 'post-experience reflective' practicums in clinical teaching.

Whichever approach is adopted, clinical teachers are faced with the immediate responsibility of preparing students for clinical practice. Although some teachers prefer to teach in the clinical setting, most recognize that there are good reasons for pre-performance practice before students use their skills in the real situation with real patients or clients. Let us examine first what is meant by 'the lab' before we explore the principles of learning and the models of nursing which could help in laboratory teaching and learning.

3.3 THE LAB IN NURSING PROGRAMMES

Activity:
The nursing lab can mean many different things to clinical teachers. From your experience, how would you describe a nursing lab? It might be helpful to ask a colleague this question and compare with your own experience.

Feedback:
The laboratory has taken many forms in nursing education. Let us examine some of them.

You may have been involved in nursing programmes where the laboratory has been the 'practical room' or the 'practice suite', and has been used mainly by students practising nursing skills to a prescribed standard before proceeding to clinical practice. In other programmes the laboratory may have been more like a tutorial or a seminar with written work and/or a presentation by students.

Certainly, the honing of procedural nursing skills in preparation for immediate practice in the clinical setting has had a long tradition in nursing programmes. Tan (1987) questions this approach, undertaken in isolation from the rest of the client care, and claims that it negates the concept of holism which is usually prominent in nursing curricula.

Laboratory work in nursing can, in modern college or university-based courses also refer to practical work in basic science laboratories. The emphasis there is on involvement in the practice of science with analysis, experimentation, interpretation and the development of basic scientific skills. In part, the nursing laboratory is analogous to the science laboratory in its aim of involving students in the practice of nursing through analysis of its theoretical background, experimentation with ideas, equipment and methods, interpretation of theory and its relation to practice, and the development of practical nursing skills.

Schweer (1972) describes the laboratory as a place where students use 'a problem-solving approach to the development of techniques in a controlled learning environment' (p. 147). The term 'laboratory method' is used by Schweer to apply to both the college workroom and to the clinical and community settings. On the other hand, Infante (1985) distinguishes between the college laboratory where there are no clients, and the clinical laboratory where students come in contact with clients. Reilly and Oermann (1985) also use the term laboratory to refer to the clinical setting, distinguishing it from the 'learning resources laboratory', which is much like the 'college laboratory' described by Infante.

Another way of identifying the laboratory in nursing is as a 'skills laboratory teaching system' (Cook and Hill, 1985). Here the emphasis is on guided practice and the system involves an elaborate set of audiovisual and computerized technology. Taylor and Cleveland (1984) use the term 'learning laboratory' to describe a similar approach to preparing students for the 'real world' of nursing. Elliott *et al.* (1982) talk about 'learning centres' comprising autotutorial resources and claim that they are not used to their potential in nursing programmes.

Infante (1985) describes the laboratory as a workshop from the Latin 'laboratorium' (p. 10), where the 'laboratory method' provides students with real experiences. The purpose of the laboratory, whether in the college or clinical setting, is

> to allow students to discover things for themselves, regardless of whether or not these things have already been discovered by others. The laboratory provides students with the opportunity to develop skill in making accurate, orderly observations. In this way they discover facts. They also discover how to learn. The importance of allowing students in the laboratory to work through problems themselves to arrive at their own conclusions cannot be overestimated. The advantages will become obvious in their subsequent practice (p. 13).

Activity:
Imagine that you have been elected by faculty members to be the co-ordinator of your nursing program. One faculty member has decided that the clinical setting rather than the lab is 'the proper place' to teach practical skills. As lab co-ordinator what will be your response?

Feedback:
After inviting the staff member concerned to talk about her/his experiences of teaching practical skills in both settings, you may wish to bring to the faculty's attention the Gomez and Gomez (1987) study which compared practice in a post-partum gynaecological unit in a general hospital with practice in the college laboratory. The study concludes that the environmental context and constraints in which the skills will be performed are important considerations. If the environmental conditions are likely to be stable and unchanging, then, practice in a lab would be indicated. However, since most nursing skills are performed in a dynamic environment with conditions which are hard to simulate in the school laboratory, the real setting allows more effective and meaningful practice of skills than does the school laboratory.

To test their assumptions the authors compared the performance of two groups of students (college lab group and patient care setting group) in measuring the blood pressure of elderly clients in a nursing home. Each group had first received identical information on blood pressure measurement, each had assembled and handled the equipment and undertaken two practice trials before being assigned randomly to one of the two groups for practice. On testing, the group that practised in the patient care setting was found to be more accurate and more confident in the basic steps of taking a blood pressure than the group who practised in the college lab.

The authors argue that students in the client care setting practice group took practice more seriously, and achieved greater mastery of the process of taking a blood pressure, than the lab practice group. Having to perform in front of clients, being concerned about safety and wanting to appear knowledgeable probably prompted the students to be better prepared for practice with 'real' patients than their counterparts who practised in the college lab first, without this pressure.

If learning to perform practical skills was the only purpose of the lab the faculty member's preference obviously would have the support of Gomez and Gomez and many others. Those who argue against learning practical skills in the reality of the clinical setting would, on the other hand, raise questions of ethical practice and patients' rights and safety.

3.4 PURPOSES OF THE LAB

Activity:
In your role as lab co-ordinator you think it is important to be clear about the purposes of the lab in your program. You decide to make a list of the purposes for your colleagues to consider. What are they?

Feedback:
Close to the top of your list you probably wrote 'getting students prepared for clinical practice', or 'giving demonstrations, supervising and assessing student practice', 'testing knowledge and skills', 'checking attitudes', 'revising theory', 'making students aware of hazards', 'calculating drug dosages', 'improving dexterity and accuracy'. Also on the list may be 'enabling self-instructional independent study or practice', 'providing practice in solving problems' and so on. Each nursing school must decide on the general purposes of the lab, usually according to the organization and design of the curriculum. In addition, individual teachers who have some of the same students for a briefing session, and the clinical practice and debriefing, may have different, or additional purposes according to the stage of learning of their group of students.

In the model of clinical teaching on which this text is based the purpose of the laboratory in the clinical learning cycle includes assisting students to:

1. understand, test and use major concepts from the theoretical programme for application to clinical practice;
2. develop skills, practical, intellectual and attitudinal as a preparation for the care of clients;
3. discover principles and develop insights through practical exercises which aim to apply basic sciences to nursing practice;
4. use an enquiry approach.

Let us examine each of these purposes.

Understand, test and use major concepts from the theoretical programme for application to clinical practice

The laboratory provides the important link between the theoretical programme and the briefing or pre-conference session before clinical practice. Even in the early stages of the programme students need to realize that their clinical skills depend to a very large extent on their knowledge base. They can then understand the rationale for procedures as well as the social, behavioural and biological principles underlying the application of skills to a number of conditions and situations.

Application of knowledge to a specific patient certainly requires that the student be familiar with the patient in order to use knowledge in the direct experience of care. However, understanding, testing and using major concepts at a general level can be undertaken in the lab. Application to a specific patient can then be made later, in the pre-conference or briefing session, immediately prior to practice in the clinical setting. For example, imagine your programme has allocated a topic such as control of infection to a lab session. The major concepts to be mastered and used by students would be derived from basic sciences, social and behavioural sciences, nursing science, and also from the students' previous practice and experience. Many types of infection could be used as the basis of exercises for students to integrate and apply their knowledge to infection control. In the briefing session to follow, a patient's specific infection and care would be the focus for the student, who now has been prepared by the more general exercises undertaken in the lab.

Develop practical and intellectual skills and shape attitudes

Laboratory teaching or the laboratory method certainly implies that students learn by actually doings things themselves. Talking about how to do things, watching others do them, or listening to others talking about how to do them is not sufficient. Moreover, the maxim

what I hear, I forget
what I see, I remember
what I do, I know

implies not an automatic response based on practice and drill but on 'knowing' in the sense of Schon's (1988) 'knowing-in-action'.

Teaching students to acquire 'knowing-in-action' is a central issue in laboratory teaching and learning. In coming to grips with the issue Tan (1987) cites Fitts and Posner's (1967) three phases of learning (cited in Singer, 1980):

Early or cognitive phase
Intermediate or associative phase
Final or autonomous phase.

In reviewing the nursing literature on this topic, Tan (1987) notes that until the final or autonomous phase is reached it is unlikely that students will be able to be effective in integrating concepts and theories of nursing with their performance of skills. Moreover, even establishing an effective relationship with a patient will be difficult for students until a pattern of performance of the skill becomes part of their memory. Only then is it possible for them to do more than one thing at once, for example, perform a surgical dressing while observing the patient's condition and reactions and while also conversing easily and purposefully. In other words perhaps skills alone should be learned first, and 'knowing-in-action' later.

Benner (1984) advocates that novices in nursing skills are given the rules to guide their performance. Is it possible that skills learned according to the rules will result in inflexible behaviour and a lack of holism? The answer is, most likely, yes, but the function of the modern nursing laboratory in the development of skills (practical and intellectual) is very different from early practical nursing training in which mastery of practical procedures was the primary aim. A level of skilled performance, which includes principles and theory, can be achieved in the laboratory and, as Benner (1984) points out, it is clearly distinguishable from the 'context-dependent judgments and skill that can be acquired only in real situations' (p. 21).

How can that be done? What implications are there for learning in the lab? The conditions for learning skills (Gagne, 1976) provide guidelines for the lab teacher in designing experiences for students to learn skills. Essentially, students must know what it is they are expected to do, know how the skill is performed, practise the skill and receive feedback on their performance. In short, the teaching skills are those of:

1. gaining attention;
2. informing the learner of the objective;
3. stimulating recall of prerequisite learning;
4. presenting stimulus material (by demonstration or problem-solving exercises);
5. providing learning guidance;
6. eliciting the performance;
7. providing feedback about performance;
8. enhancing retention and transfer.

Development of dexterity, practice in assembling and dismantling equipment, making errors and identifying how to correct them, recognizing improvement in one's own performance, and giving feedback to colleagues in a simulated exercise, all require space, time, equipment and teacher interest and guidance.

Discussing lab teaching in biological sciences Hegarty-Hazel (1988, p. 56) offers the following as a guide for lab teachers:

1. provide students with a satisfying rationale for learning the techniques (e.g. use with patients or important prerequisite)

2. help students understand the logic or overview of the skills routine and to understand links with related perceptual skills and knowledge

3. provide opportunities for practice and feedback to improve the accuracy, speed and quality of the component-part skills

4. take account of the fact that, once mastered, technical skills are well remembered and retained and they continue to improve with practice.

Practice in thinking while acting is another dimension to be included in laboratory learning of skills. Tan (1987) shows how the teaching methods of 'guided discovery' and problem-solving prompt the student to think through the purposes of the specific activity or procedure, not in isolation, but within a nursing process exercise. This is important as the student can then learn to question the adequacy of the method for achieving the purpose and to criticize the rationale for the use of the procedure in the first place. Access to readings and relevant research reports adds to the student's background information. Armed with principles and theories from the coursework the student is well prepared to think-in-action while learning the skill. However, students need considerable guidance from teachers to enable them to practise thinking and reflecting-in-action. While reflection is usually associated with the debriefing stage of the clinical learning cycle, exercises designed to help students reflect on their performance can be introduced in the lab.

Shaping attitudes, the third component associated with learning practical skills, should also be part of lab learning. Although an artificial setting, the lab can show desirable models of behaviour through role models, demonstration or video, attitudes of caring, sensitivity, responsibility, honesty and reliability to name a few. Similarly, role play recorded on video and played back can be a powerful tool to raise students' awareness of unacceptable as well as desirable attitudes.

Discover principles and develop insights through practical exercises which aim to apply basic sciences to nursing practice

Is it possible for students to develop skills in critical thinking through exercises in the lab? Most clinical teachers would want students to achieve practical skills within the context of total care and to question the methods and the rationale underlying interventions and procedures. Most would also support the use of the lab as an integrating mechanism to draw theory and practice closer together. Curriculum objectives often require that students integrate and apply the concepts, principles and theories from the sciences (relevant physical, biological, social) and in some cases, also spiritual approaches, to clinical practice. Examples such as the following can be found in most programmes:

1. Apply relevant theoretical concepts and principles in the performance of selected nursing care activities for individuals across the age continuum and in different disorder categories.
2. Synthesize knowledge from applied and behavioural sciences with nursing theory as a base for nursing practice.

How effective is the lab in assisting students to reach these objectives? It is probably not too wide of the mark to suggest that clinical teachers have had more comfort in appealing to the biological base of nursing practice than to the social and behavioural science base. Although many reasons can be advanced, the historical one is probably the most valid. Certainly, nursing inherited a firm foundation from the almost universal applicability of principles from the basic sciences. The precedent set by curricula in the past (in most health professions) where disease and its biological, physical and chemical origin overshadowed its behavioural base influenced teaching in both theoretical and practical components of the course (White *et al.*, 1988b). There are good reasons, therefore, for lab teaching to draw upon the major concepts from the range of relevant sciences, including social and behavioural, so that students learn to discover principles and develop insights into nursing practice.

In the clinical learning cycle, the lab is the focus for application of sciences to practice in a general sense, independent of the problems of specific patients. A method of approach can be learned in the lab, but it is in the briefing and debriefing sessions where the actual context and particular patient's problem are the focus. In that respect the concepts from the social and behavioural sciences are likely to be especially relevant. As a nurse with a social and behavioural science background points out:

> Principle and concepts (of nursing) have universal applicability but nursing *behaviours* are contextually derived according to the individual nursing environment (Cottier, 1986 quoted in *Windows onto Worlds* 1987, p. 158).

It is worth remembering that nursing practice is more than getting the theory in place and using it to improve practice. Learning nursing practice also involves the development of the student as a reasoning professional practitioner who can derive insights from practice. While it is true that reasoning skills and the use of abstractions are developed over time and during experience, there is merit in encouraging new students in the lab, to reflect on their own reasoning processes. Students can be helped to see that there is richness in the challenging complexity underlying the concrete practical skills so often taken for granted.

Use the skills of enquiry

Most nursing courses now include the nursing process as a way of teaching problem solving and enquiry skills. Unfortunately, the nursing process is now so much a part of courses that the 'process' is in danger of becoming a technique rather than a thoughtful way of interlinking observations with the thinking processes of assessment, decision-making, planning, action and evaluation.

Courses which have chosen a problem-based curriculum have developed enquiry methods which are integral to lab and tutorial teaching and which become the students' clinical practice mode.

3.5 DESIGN OF THE LAB – PHYSICAL FACILITIES

What physical facilities are required for a modern nursing lab?

Activity:
As lab co-ordinator you have been appointed by the Dean to chair a committee to suggest the physical facilities of a new lab. What information about lab designs will your committee seek?

Feedback:
You could refer to the lab designs in the early nursing programmes of community college programmes in USA as a starting point. These programmes considered the lab to be critical in the preparation of students for clinical practice. For example, the concise prescription of Montag (1951) for the requirements of a lab is as relevant to

today's teaching as it was forward-looking then. It is interesting to note that contrary to trends at that time, a simulated ward is not recommended. Instead

> The laboratory should be so equipped that the students will have opportunity to see demonstrations of nursing techniques and to secure skill in the execution of these techniques. The equipment required should be like that found in the hospital, home, and other agencies in which the student will have clinical experience. The laboratory should be large enough to permit individual practice units and be equipped with adequate materials to allow a number of students to practise at the same time. A unit completely equipped for demonstration should be included. Dressing rooms, lockers, and storage facilities are essential parts of the laboratory (p. 101).

Labs of the 1980s and 1990s not only simulate a hospital ward but a client's home as well. Convertible lounges or bedrooms to reflect different economic and social conditions are simulated so that students practise in as realistic an environment as possible. Typical bathrooms with problems of wheelchair access provide for practice of strategies which are alternatives to hospital methods and confront students with the need to improvise and initiate solutions in collaboration with the client. Teachers in programmes such as Deakin University in Victoria and the South Australian Institute of Technology (South Australia) use such simulated facilities and combine learning of concepts from the theoretical component of the course with application to realistic nursing practice problems in typical client surroundings.

The argument in support of simulated wards and domestic settings claims that a learning experience should be structured to resemble as nearly as possible the actual setting of future practice. While this is an important principle for predictive testing of performance its validity for learning professional practice is doubtful. Realism in the practice situation is only one aspect of the design of the learning task and although it is arguably important, questions of what students learn beyond the manipulation of equipment and the reduction of hazards in the environment need to be raised. In the light of the purposes of your particular lab you may wish to consider whether a duplication of the clinical or community setting is really necessary.

The idea of presenting the student with a faithful replica of a ward dates from the era where students were employees and needed to practise ward duties in the 'preliminary training school'. Familiarity with the fixed environment of ward furniture was desirable and was used in the early stages of training. Once the students' introductory period was completed it is doubtful whether it was ever used as a ward again by those students. Now that students are learners in academic institutions with a planned programme of laboratory exercises sequenced to complement the theoretical programme, the necessity of the traditional design of the practice room, or laboratory, should be questioned. If you have ever tried to have students undertake group or individual exercises which do not involve a bed or a client, you will agree that the resources of a simulated ward are not ideal. Group discussion rooms or small rooms for practice with resources appropriate to the exercises are an alternative where students can work on problems to assist them to integrate their knowledge and check out their understanding with their colleagues or with a teacher.

Several questions may help you to identify the proportion of learning that could, and should, occur in the lab.

1. What learning experiences do not require a patient in order for skills to be learned?
2. What skills can be learned in the college or school laboratory before requiring performance in the actual setting?
3. What learning experiences can only occur in the context of actual practice?
4. At what stage is it desirable that those learning experiences occur?
5. In what situation is it educationally and practically desirable for the learning experiences to occur? In the client's home or in a nursing home or hospital with beds, patients and equipment?

Summary

If the learning in the lab is to comprise skills, both practical and intellectual then equipment resembling what students will use in clinical will be required and sufficient space and supplies for the number of students in each lab session to use comfortably. It is desirable that all the equipment is movable so that the different purposes of the lab can be accommodated.

If the learning is to promote critical thinking then the lab needs additional space to serve as a resources bay with reading materials, sequenced problem exercises and space for examining and/or constructing aids for clients or designing alternatives to current equipment or products.

3.6 MANAGING THE LAB SESSION

Activity:
In your role as lab co-ordinator you have been asked by new teachers for advice about the management of lab sessions. What suggestions will you give them?

Feedback:
Management of lab sessions often consists simply of preparing the equipment, giving the demonstration and supervising students' practice. Certainly, that is one part of the lab and expertise in demonstrating is an important teaching skill. There are, of course, many other components of the lab to be managed so that students are active and involved, and the lab work is relevant to their current progress in learning. The sequence of lab learning must also be managed so that it is meaningful and students can retain and retrieve necessary information. It is also important that students are encouraged and supported.

The lab session itself can be thought of as a small group session with up to 20 students.

Lab teaching is probably one of the most difficult teaching and learning sessions to organize and manage. Romanini (1988) has devised a model of the teacher-manager which can be applied to many aspects of teaching and is admirably suited to lab teaching. 'The Teacher-Manager (T-M) Model' identifies three stages in the management of a learning program. They are (pp. 218–219):

1. *Preparation.* This stage includes those activities which it is desirable for the teacher/manager to perform, in order to assist learners in the preparation of a learning task.
2. *Implementation.* This stage includes those functions of a teacher/manager which are associated with encouraging students to accomplish the learning task.
3. *Evaluation.* This stage involves the teacher/manager in conducting evaluation of the learning programme in conjunction with the students.

As Figure 3.2 shows, each stage has several phases. Romanini's model provides a step-by-step pathway with emphasis on the stage of preparation to ensure that planning to meet students' learning

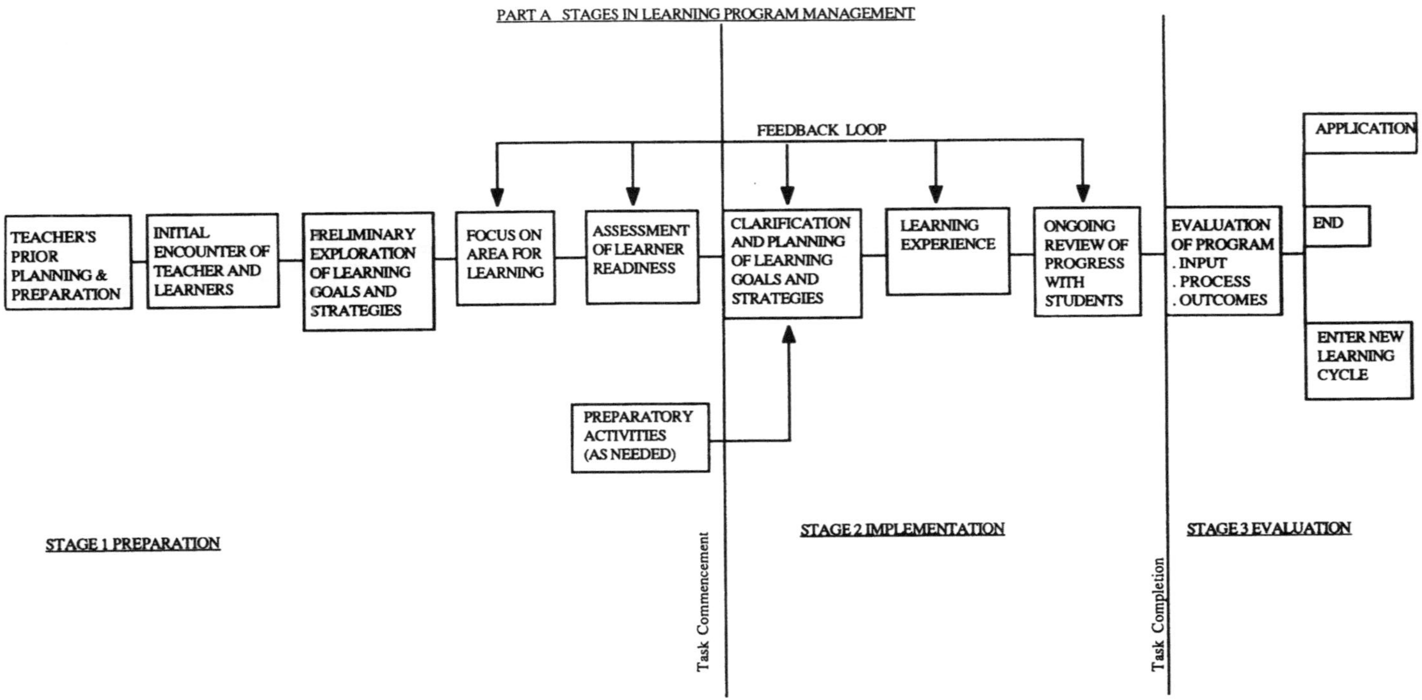

Figure 3.2 Teacher–manager model.

Source: Romanini (1988).

needs is given sufficient thought. The teacher-manager role is built on the premise that if the lab is planned, structured and organized to maximize student learning and performance, the teacher's role is predominantly concerned with assisting students to identify their individual learning stage and pace and organizing resources for maximizing self-directed learning and encouraging self-assessment.

Planning the lab

Detailed planning is essential so that students are given sufficient direction, facilitation and supervision. Planning will include availability and accessibility of resources according to the number of students and staff, testing of the equipment to be used in demonstrations (and return demonstrations), assembling of diagrams, posters, charts and handouts, and arranging seating for students so that observation of the demonstration and participation in questions and discussions is facilitated.

Organizing the facilities

There are many ways in which lab facilities can be designed; for example, according to the objectives of the programme, the purpose of the particular lab and the learning stage of the students. Here are a few examples:

The lab may be set up as a number of different stations around the room, each one with a set of problems, questions or activities to be completed. Sets of equipment and directions are supplied for each station. The class, in groups of three or four (client, student, observer(s)), then work together on the tasks at each station, and at a pre-determined time, move on to the next, until the round is completed. For example, Figure 3.3 shows a simple room arrangement and examples of problems and activities. The teacher as resource person circulates among the stations. Student self-testing and testing by peers is encouraged, followed by assessment of 'critical' areas of performance supervised by the teacher.

Planning for this type of lab is time-consuming and detailed. You would need to weigh up whether the results in terms of student motivation and performance of the tasks as well as understanding the application of the associated principles were sufficient to justify your time and effort. The advantages are in active, peer-supported learning, problem-solving and practice and in building confidence.

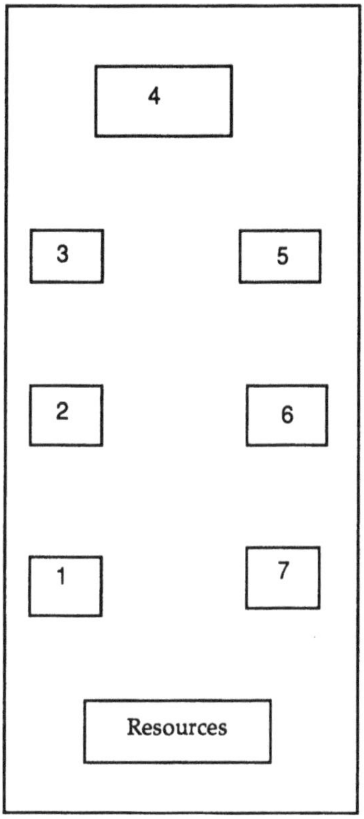

LAB SESSION: OPTHALMIC NURSING

1. Experiencing perceptual deprivation - trust walk and questions to identify implications of deprivation

2. Identifying effects of social deprivation and recognition of compensatory behaviour. Identifying appropriate nursing actions and sensitivities

3. Pre-test of structure and function of visual system by completion of test diagrams. Self-assessment.
Testing visual acuity.
Testing light reflex

4. Observing and examining the eye, conjunctiva and lids, describing results giving and receiving feedback on skill from colleagues

5. Instillation of drops and revising action of medications

6. Practising eye treatments and analysing side effects, hazards and designing protective measures.

7. Short post-test, self assessment and plan for follow-up.

Figure 3.3 Lab layout and examples of problems and activities at work stations.

Any inactive 'waiting' time in labs should be avoided through effective planning to prevent students becoming bored and apathetic.

Problem-based learning labs require extensive preparation of stimulus material such as a 'problem box' or 'situation improvement packages' (Ryan, 1989). Other programmes use pre- and post-tests as stimulus material and for self-assessment and indication of progress.

Access to the lab

Infante (1985) notes that students are not always motivated to practise skills at the precise times the laboratory may be open and suggests that access to the college laboratory be available during a wider range of hours than is usually the case. Some of the time could be for students to practise by themselves; at other times when students are requesting feedback or guidance, teachers also need to be available during a wider range of hours.

3.7 MODELS OF LAB TEACHING AND LEARNING

Activity:
Your Dean has asked for examples of the models of laboratory teaching before making a decision on the new lab. What will your committee present?

Feedback:
Clinical teaching which requires low student/teacher ratios is therefore expensive. For this reason efficient and effective use of laboratory teaching is a priority and considerable attention has been paid to developing innovative models and strategies.

The idea of 'laboratory teaching' comes from the work of Dewey (1916) who believed that 'learning by doing' together with solving problems provided a type of learning ideal for understanding the relevance of science to professional practice (Infante, 1985; Schweer, 1972). Most of the models of lab teaching include the two components of active involvement and problem-solving. Traditional exercises and demonstrations have given way to laboratory teaching comprising many different methods. In a survey of methods in laboratory teaching in tertiary science courses the following eight approaches were found (Boud *et al.*, 1978). Laboratory teaching in nursing programmes have adopted most of these models, either separately, or in various combinations.

Models of laboratory teaching in tertiary science courses, adapted for nursing labs

Keller plan or personalized system of instruction (PSI). Independent learning labs where nursing students work at their own pace, and at times which suit their study and clinical programmes, have been used to provide opportunities for students to gain competence and speed in practical skills.

Audio-tutorial method (A-T). Carrels, audiovisual equipment and study/practice guides, enable students to work independently. Students view a video or listen to an audiotape while following an accompanying manual, answer a pre-practice quiz and then proceed to a skills lab for practice and finally, for assessment.

Computer assisted learning (CAL). Where these expensive computer programs are used as an instructional tool together with videodisc, the student is taken through a nursing practice situation, to which he/she responds with a suggested action, is given feedback and finally directed to perform an activity, report on it, and enter the result into the computer. If unsatisfactory, further feedback, practice and comments are entered before the student proceeds to the next lab sequence.

Learning aids laboratory (LAL). Additional learning opportunities are provided in these labs to enable students to gain skills and knowledge in special activities normally outside the usual programme. An example would be the skills associated with specialist areas in clinical nursing where all students would not necessarily gain experience during the course, nor would all clinical teachers possess appropriate specialist clinical skills. These labs are sometimes called 'clinical workshops'. Clinicians conduct the labs which are usually intensive over at least one day, and more usually one week, so that students have time to observe demonstrations, ask questions, become familiar with equipment, practise skills on each other and receive feedback on knowledge and skills.

Modular laboratory. A direct link between the theoretical programme and the clinical setting is provided through laboratory modules dealing with separate sequences of learning, complete in each module. A learning package is provided for students and a teacher's guide for the clinical teachers. For example, a module in the maternal and child health programme on, say, post-natal care, would contain a summary of material from the theoretical component of the course, followed by a summary of the appropriate nursing roles, functions and skills, a case study used as an application exercise in the lab, and finally a clinical assignment with objectives, directions and guidelines for practice and assessment.

Integrated laboratory. Several disciplines combine to teach, for example, physics concepts through practical nursing problems. The principles of force, gravitation, torque and levers can be applied to practical nursing activities such as observing body alignment, positioning in illness, bedmaking and traction.

In a fully integrated lab, principles from biological and physical sciences and social and behavioural concepts and nursing science are applied to clinical states (such as immobility, dependency, restlessless, stress) and after working on understanding the underlying concepts, students identify the appropriate skills for nursing practice in the lab. An example of an integrated lab applied to the clinical state of immobility would result in practical care of clients immobilized for various causes or treatments, together with skills of observation, communication, assessment of health status and the design of care plans.

Project work. Community health nursing projects, commenced in the lab and continued in community agencies or the client's home are an example.

Participation in research. Although not common in undergraduate nursing labs, the experience of involvement in a clinical research study enables senior students to apply the enquiry skills learned earlier in the programme to the research process.

Models of laboratory teaching in nursing – developed by clinical teachers

As well as adapting models from other professional fields, clinical teachers in nursing have developed labs to meet their special needs and approaches to learning and practice.

Skills learning laboratory simulation system. An interesting nursing lab is described by Cook and Hill (1985). Their successful 'skills learning laboratory simulation system' began as a way of reducing the stress of new nursing students in the clinical setting. In addition, in the safety of a controlled environment the students' competence could be determined and clinical faculty preceptors would know what knowledge and dexterity should be expected from students entering the clinical area.

The instructional strategy used is a 'partner system', consisting of pairs of students working together. This is a means of providing support and 'low-pressure peer review' as well as enabling each learner to be both 'patient' and 'nurse' as they progress through the skills lab system. A set of skill modules is supplied consisting of audiovisuals and written material which the students must view and read before taking a 'brief post-module quiz'. Immediate feedback is given and the student partners proceed to the practice area following the guide in the module. They practise first, and request assistance from a faculty member if their own attempts are unsuccessful.

Importantly, the skills are introduced concurrently with the theory students receive in the lecture programme and practice sites are chosen so that application of theory and skill will be facilitated.

Simulated lab. Infante (1985, Chapter 5) gives a detailed account of how simulation can be a model for laboratory teaching. A simulated lab provides excellent opportunities for providing a setting as near as possible to reality. Infante gives examples of case analysis, games, written simulations, role-playing, audio-visual resources such as films, tapes and simulators, and lastly, but most importantly, the simulated client or patient.

Clinical skills collaborative workshop. Short, intensive workshops may be designed at regular intervals so that senior students who are nearing graduation can have opportunities to revise and practise with, and to learn from, clinical staff of specialty departments. The programme of the workshops is directed by the students' needs and usually is conducted in the college lab, but may be in a special department if complex equipment is involved. These workshops combine several purposes: mastery of complex skills; allaying anxiety about impending reponsibilities as a registered nurse; enhancing collaborative and co-operative relationships across clinical and education institutions and between students and registered nurses.

3.8 CURRICULUM DESIGN AND LAB TEACHING AND LEARNING

Activity:
In many nursing programmes the curriculum has been developed to reflect the views of the faculty on how students learn and how nursing should be practised. Take a few moments to peruse the curriculum of your programme for indications of the preferred approaches to teaching and learning in the lab.

Feedback:
You will probably agree that this is an important question which needs Faculty-wide discussion. If we believe, with Stevens (1979), that the curriculum does indeed influence teaching then deciding on a *modus operandi* is an important faculty development issue.

How does a problem-based learning programme affect teaching in the lab?

Perhaps the most influential in structuring lab teaching and learning, the problem-based nursing curriculum presents a radically different picture from traditional structures for teacher and learner in the lab, tutorial and in clinical practice. Andersen (1990a) reports the progress of problem-based learning at one nursing school and reports the success of 'contextualizing' student learning. Contextualizing learning implies structuring a learning environment that is 'action-based', is more relevant to students as it mirrors the situation in which they practise, and in addition strengthens the cycle of theory–practice–theory. The key aspects of problem-based learning are knowledge structured for use in clinical contexts; the development of an effective clinical reasoning process and effective self-directed learning skills; and the increase of motivation for learning.

What difference does this make to learning in the laboratory?

Because problem-based courses are organized around problems it follows that learning will be focused on integration of subjects rather than separate areas which are then integrated in clinical practice. Ryan and Little (1989) explain the approach in these terms:

> The focus of this integration is on actual clinical cases in the form of SIPS (Situation Improvement Packages). Thus a student may be required to "nurse" a "patient" with a disturbance of activities of daily living associated with gastro-intestinal dysfunction and in the process will be required to explore content which would traditionally be organised under curriculum areas such as Anatomy and Physiology (in this instance in the gastro-intestinal tract), Behavioural Studies (eg. the concept of "body image" and the young person's reaction to the need for a colostomy), Practice Principles and Skills (eg. stomatherapy) and so on. The important point to note is that traditional content is not overlooked; rather it is explored in the integrated context of an actual clinical case.

This example shows that all the purposes of laboratory learning (pp. 39–43 above) will be met, but not through the usual 'learning laboratory' concept. Indeed another model is used. This is a problem-based tutorial with situation improvement packages, and access to practice principles and skills sessions relevant to the package being learned.

Ryan and Little (1989) expands the notion of problem-based learning to show how students are immersed in the patient's problem:

> When "nursing" the "patient" the students are required to respond to cues, prioritise the patient's needs and problems, generate and test hypotheses, make clinical judgements and plan and evaluate appropriate care. By focusing on a patient situation, the students' judgments and actions are always in response to a particular set of conditions which have a unique combination of elements. While it is true that the students will be guided by rules, these are practised in the context of the situation, so that it is the situation which determines the judgments and actions, not the rules. Although these learning experiences are simulations, their approximation of reality is enhanced by the set of actual chart data, audio-visual representations and simulated patients. The classroom is contextualised; the learning experiences consist of a repertoire of concrete examples such as described by Benner and Schon as the basis of practitioner knowledge.

In a number of nursing programmes, problem-solving labs are used, although the curriculum is not designed as a problem-based course. The encouragement of problem-solving skills is achieved through a variety of designs of lab learning. An example in a programme using the activities of daily living as a conceptual base would be a lab starting with concepts from the theoretical programme dealing with muscular dysfunction (e.g. relevant anatomy and physiology, social and behavioural science, nursing science). The students would then work on a problem-list of relevant conditions, the task being to identify the nursing care required. Students would then interview a person with muscular dysfunction (either simulated or real) and identify what modifications of clinical skills would be required for specific procedures. The equipment would be identified and students would practise the required skills.

Other labs aimed at self-direction and autonomy use a problem-solving learning contract. In a unit of study (for example, Maternal and Child Health), the concepts from the theoretical programme related to physiological, psychological and social changes during pregnancy are revised in the lab. The skills practised in the lab include interviewing, urinalysis, taking blood pressure, dietary assessment, health education techniques. A contract focusing on antenatal care is then drawn up by the student, negotiated with the clinical teacher and completed by the student in a community health centre.

How does a competency-based curriculum affect teaching and learning in the lab?

The history of competency-based nursing programmes can be traced through a number of stages of curriculum development. Attempts to integrate curriculum content and relate theoretical knowledge to clinical problems have used a 'competencies approach'. The knowledge background and understanding of nursing practice necessary to achieve each competency can be traced to relevant areas in the curriculum.

Other programmes have been committed to the 'definition of all educational goals in terms of explicit behavioural descriptions of what a person is able to do once an educational activity has been mastered' (Monjan and Gassner, 1979, p. 4). When competencies are framed in this way some of the objections raised about the global nature of competencies are overcome. Pratt (1989) is concerned that the broad expression of competencies cloaks the relationship of the competency with the psychomotor skills students are expected to perform. 'It is the very global nature of the term "competencies" which has masked the specificity of subsumed skills and militated against their identification – an identification which would appear crucial in terms of preparing qualified practitioners who can demonstrate the requisite behavioural repertoire' (p. 20). The point is that a misuse of precious learning and experience time could result if the lab were to be structured for learning skills which are not necessary in the initial professional performance of the beginning practitioner.

Some competency-based programmes have taken 'global' competencies, such as contained in the New South Wales Nursing Registration Board's Guidelines for Curricula (1984). For example:

> The graduate nurse should be able to:
>
> . . . plan and provide appropriate care to meet the needs of the individual, the family or group

and the related objectives:

> In developing this competency the student nurse should be able to:
>
> . . . demonstrate a problem-solving approach to the planning of individual care;
>
> . . . develop care plans;
>
> . . . demonstrate an ability to assist in meeting the individual's physiological and psychosocial needs;

> ... apply principles of nursing and related sciences to the practice of nursing.

The specific skills required to perform the competency are then extracted.

The skills are practised in a Nursing Practice Workshop prior to a period of clinical practice. Teaching and learning in the lab is directed toward mastering the skills (practical and intellectual). The knowledge base underlying the skills must be mastered as well as the skills. In briefing and clinical practice sessions the clinical teacher helps students to realize how the skills and knowledge mastered in the lab relate to the total competency. As the students' level of learning increases they are able to apply the competency in many different situations and contexts.

How does a curriculum designed as concept-based affect teaching and learning in the lab?

Ausubel's notion of meaningful learning is based on the premise that when content is presented according to an organized set of concepts and principles students' cognitive structures are modified so that retention and retrieval of information is enhanced. Ausubel claims that 'advance organizers' act as a bridge between knowledge learners have stored and new learning to be acquired. The 'advance organizer' prompts appropriate parts of the learner's cognitive structure and promotes readiness to 'connect' with new knowledge and/or experience. The relevance for clinical teaching is clear. If students have acquired a set of concepts from a curriculum built on a conceptual framework, their cognitive structures have been influenced so that meaningful learning occurs as the concepts are developed, extended and applied.

A programme built on a conceptual framework for nursing practice is reported by Kermode (1986). The framework of the programme at Riverina-Murray Institute of Higher Education (RMIHE) drew on the work of Henderson (1966), Roy (1970) and Roper (1980). Three broad constructs, Humankind, Health and Nursing Practice, were chosen and the concepts in each identified. Interwoven with the construct of Health were activities of daily living such as:

> those related to comfort: maintaining safety and security; maintaining hygiene and body warmth; avoiding pain; achieving rest

> those related to normal body functions: breathing, eating and drinking; eliminating wastes; mobilizing, sensing and perceiving
>
> those related to personal growth and fulfilment: expressing sexuality; working; playing and creative expression; communicating; learning; expressing emotions, including grieving (p. 30).

Within the construct of Nursing Practice, analysis of the nursing activities which directly affect clients resulted in the identification of three major concepts, which in turn revealed a series of sub-concepts. The major concepts were: Promotion; Supporting; Intervening.

The staff at RMIHE integrated the concepts of the nursing process into the final conceptual framework for nursing practice. This development resulted in a flow chart which directed students through the major constructs and concepts as they applied them to practice through the use of the nursing process.

3.9 LEARNING PROBLEMS AND TEACHING SKILLS

By now it is clear that the type of curriculum, the stage of the students, and the purposes and design of the lab all influence teaching and learning in the lab. Obviously, there is no one way to teach or to learn. There are, however, principles of teaching and established methods for teaching which should be accessible in foundation educational texts. Principal authorities on skills learning are Gagne (1976); Fits and Posner (1967); Singer (1980); for teaching problem-solving, Barrows (1988); and for the teaching skill of demonstration in nursing see, for example, Schweer (1972); Ewan and White (1984); Infante (1985); de Tornyay (1982).

Since demonstration is such a frequent teaching method in a nursing lab, it is worthwhile including a framework of questions clinical teachers can use to guide the planning of a demonstration (Figure 3.4).

In this text we are identifying those teaching skills which the clinical teacher uses and which are additional to the skills utilized in the classroom or in small groups. That is not to say that the usual teaching skills such as questioning, explaining, reinforcing, rewarding, responding, interacting and giving feedback (Turney *et al.*, 1973, 1975) are dismissed in clinical teaching. Certainly they are all used. In this text each section of the clinical learning cycle will deal with the specific teaching skills appropriate for that segment of the cycle.

1. What are the purposes or objectives of your demonstration?

If your objectives require students to be able to perform the task you are demonstrating then you must also provide opportunities for practice and feedback.

2. What can you do to increase the students' involvement in the demonstration?

Almost by definition a demonstration causes the audience to be passive. Learners learn better when they are actively involved. You should therefore plan your demonstration so that students are required to become involved in it in some way rather than to just watch. Ask some students to help, some to act as observers, provide written handouts and questions to guide students' thinking and observations, stop the demonstration at suitable points for questions and discussion and make sure that every student has a good view of what is happening.

3. What are the main points you want to make in the demonstration?

Begin the demonstration by telling students briefly what you are about to do and summarise the main points they should watch for. You could choose some of the students to note down their observations at those key points and you should also point these out as they occur. By providing such a 'road map' through the demonstration you can ensure that students do not get lost in the technical details which might be likely to distract their attention. At the end of the demonstration ask the students to summarise the lessons learned.

4. What resources will you require to carry out the demonstration?

Obviously you will assemble and check all the necessary technical equipment or materials for your demonstration beforehand. It is also worth thinking about whether any additional resources such as diagrams or handouts will help the students to get the most benefit from the demonstration. For example you could provide an observation check-list which requires the students to fill in their observations against certain questions or headings on the sheet.

5. Is the relevance of the demonstration clear?

Since demonstrations can be quite complex and time-consuming you should be sure that the demonstration is actually necessary for the achievement of your objectives. You should also make sure that students understand the relevance of the demonstration to what they are learning to do. Otherwise they may find it confusing or boring.

6. Have you provided opportunities for supervised practice and return demonstration?

Once you are satisfied with the students' level of skill and understanding of the basic principles applied to clinical practice then the students can be moved on through the next level of clinical education which is practice under supervision in a real setting, most often, the ward or community centre.

Figure 3.4 Characteristics of an effective demonstration.

Source: Ewan and White (1984, pp. 110–111).

Just as there is no one way to teach or to learn, there is no general prescription for solving the problems of clinical teaching which may, and do, arise. What can be said is that awareness of possible problems early in the clinical learning cycle (that is, in the lab) will reduce their occurrence later in clinical practice. Some examples of clinical teaching and learning problems are given in this chapter. The problems were highlighted during a project to identify clinical teaching skills (White *et al.*, 1988(a)). They are:

1. overcoming students' lack of experience;
2. including the patient in the learning triad;
3. intervening to give correction or feedback;
4. applying theory to practice;
5. closing the learning/practice gap.

These problems are not exclusively the domain of lab teaching and learning; they occur in all stages of the clinical learning cycle. The teacher's role in assisting students to overcome these problems involves a number of clinical teaching skills in each stage of the clinical learning cycle. Let us consider how the problems can be addressed by the clinical teacher in the lab.

Problem 1. Overcoming students' lack of experience

Activity:
Most new students have had little experience of the clinical environment in which they will be expected to perform. How can the clinical teacher assist these students in the lab? To identify some of the problems, try asking your students to draw a simple picture of the most important (or frightening, or exciting, or unexpected) aspect of the clinical setting for them and invite them to compare their perceptions with others in the group.

Feedback:
Exercises like this in the lab can help new students to think through their perceptions. Not infrequently, popular media images influence students' approach to their new experiences and an interesting discussion can result from inviting students to trace the origin of their impressions. This may be useful in reducing the distortion (if any) in their perceptions. Nevertheless, new students are 'captives' of their previous conditioning and need time before they can come to terms with the realities of clinical practice. The first step the teacher can take is to recognize that over-confident or, alternatively, timid behaviour is related to the unfamiliarity of the student with the complex environment in which nursing takes place. Equally, the level of performance expected of new students is also among their concerns.

New challenges pose questions of the meaning of new experiences and raise doubts for students about their abilities and self-worth. Students' concerns are many, but particularly, as beginners, their attempts in mastering practical skills, and in trying to interact satisfactorily, can leave them feeling frustrated and ineffective. New students, inexperienced in initiating a conversation with a sick or disabled person, may hide their anxieties with a display of confidence, or at the other extreme, be blunt or abrasive. The effect on the patient is more troubling when issues of the patient role, sick role, age role, ethnic, status or power roles are considered.

What can the lab teacher do? In conjunction with the early lab classes of skill learning, the teacher can give informed support based on the recognition of the beginning students' problems. (Remembering one's own experiences as a new student brings interesting and sensitive perceptions to the students' situation.)

All students need concrete information about standards of performance; new students are particularly vulnerable and they should be given clear expectations of the level of performance demanded. Establishing standards of, for example, accuracy, dexterity, asepsis and comfort, can be satisfactorily accomplished in the lab, and followed by adequate practice, enables the over-confident and brash as well as the timid and withdrawn to come to terms with an objective measure of their own performance.

Most teachers would agree that students are more assured when they have mastered a few essential practical skills and that they are then able to be less anxious about interacting with patients. However, in practice, these events are usually not sequential but intertwined. Practice in the lab needs to reflect the clinical practice situation and the teacher needs to encourage interaction of students in a simulated clinical problem context.

In summary, to assist students to overcome their lack of experience, the teaching skills in the lab include the following:

1. *Recognizing students' concern*: allow time to discuss fears, expectations, hopes.
2. *Giving informed support*: acknowledge newness; indicate willingness for further individual discussions; provide details of available assistance.
3. *Establishing standards of performance*: demonstrate method of attaining accuracy, dexterity, comfort, etc. Give feedback on students' performance.
4. *Encouraging interaction*: introduce simple communication exer-

cises; provide simulated 'patients' for introductory conversations with students as they perform tasks to established standards.

Problem 2. Including the patient in the learning triad

Activity:
In the busy activities of clinical teaching the patient is often excluded. Ask a colleague to observe and to give feedback on how you include the patient in a clinical teaching session.

Feedback:
It is usual for the student to be the focus of a clinical learning session. This often results in the teacher and the student interacting while the patient remains passive. Several consequences can follow: the students adopt the teacher's role-model as acceptable for their own performance; the patient becomes an object for the student's learning; the teacher retains a demonstrating or lecturing style and uses correct but unnecessarily complex technical language.

In the lab, demonstrations of a clinical procedure are excellent occasions for showing how the patient can be included. Rather than a simple 'good bedside manner' what is meant by including the patient is a change in approach to teaching. Finding ways to make explanations explicit to the patient as well as the students; obtaining feedback from both students and patient; and using language understandable to the patient as well as the student, are all involved.

Role play in the lab is an excellent way of demonstrating that the patient is learning as well as receiving nursing care; just as the students themselves are learning as well as giving care. Sometimes, in the real workplace, what is learned is far from ideal and can reinforce the patient's feeling of powerlessness. The student–patient encounter, when interactive and reciprocal, supports both student and patient and provides both with the knowledge they need. What the teacher can do in the lab is demonstrate how to go further than the courtesies of introductions, asking for permission for, and giving information about the care or treatment, and thanking the patient for contributing to student learning. The teacher can, in addition, deliberately invite the patient to take part by asking questions, giving suggestions and feedback.

The approach of the clinical teacher is more aligned to the notion of 'incidental learning' than to a more formal 'patient education' or 'health education' programme. The teaching skills are therefore opportunistic.

1. *Enhancing the patient's understanding of the condition or treatment*: prompt students to put explanations in everyday words.
2. *Using occasions for encouraging the patient's self-confidence in asking questions*:
   (a) allow a particular time for questions from the patient as well as the student;
   (b) give equal attention and interest to both;
   (c) listen for the 'unasked' question;
   (d) answer questions from both patient and student openly and honestly; or
   (e) give reasons why some questions cannot or should not be answered at that time and make special arrangements to resume at a later time.
3. *Seeking feedback on the clarity of explanations or directions about treatment or care*: encourage students to ask non-threatening questions to confirm that their explanations were understood and appropriate.
4. *Stimulating interest in self-care*:
   (a) raise ideas of how the patient can become more involved in own care;
   (b) ask for suggestions from both patient and student;
   (c) offer further opportunities to pursue individual approaches.

Students generally learn about patients, their illness or problem, disease, signs and symptoms, treatment, prognosis and so on. Realizing that they can also learn from patients is important in widening the scope of knowledge beyond the actual clinical assignment to the social and behavioural environment factors important to individual patients. Patients usually are unaware that apart from the study of their condition or illness they can, personally, contribute to the student's learning. In turn they can learn from the student's questions and explanations that protecting their future health involves more than the resolution of the immediate problem or disease condition.

Problem 3. Intervening to give correction or feedback

Activity:
An important part of clinical teaching is correcting errors and giving information so that performance can be improved. When an action needs correction during clinical practice the teacher must intervene. Think back to when a teacher 'took over' from you during clinical practice. What was your reaction? Make a list of the behaviours of the teacher you most admired and those you deplored.

Feedback:

Many nurses have memories of unfortunate instances of correction given harshly in front of the patient, without feedback to show how to improve. Anxiety, fear and uncertainty of how to proceed were common complications and most would agree their learning and their performance regressed. Although this is a problem for the clinical practice session where the patient is present, the clinical teacher and students need to address the problem well before the event. If the performance threatens the patient's safety and well-being there is no alternative. The student must be stopped there and then. However, the situation is often not so clear cut and the clinical teacher is faced with deciding whether the performance can continue so that the student is not embarrassed in front of the patient and the patient's confidence in the student is retained. Feedback can then be given following the performance. On the other hand, there is a dilemma in deciding which has priority, the patient's needs or the student's learning. In each different situation the clinical teacher needs to decide whether to intervene, how to intervene and give feedback in such a way as to benefit both patient and student.

How do clinical teachers resolve the dilemma? There are two aspects; intervention and feedback. These two aspects can be addressed in the lab between teacher and students. When, and how to intervene can be negotiated with the understanding that there will be occasions when performance in clinical practice must be stopped, but in a way that will not alarm the patient. Appropriate signals to the student, determined in the lab and practised during supervision of clinical procedures, can be contracted satisfactorily between students and teacher. The student is then aware of the necessity to cease treatment, or to change what is being done, or alternatively, to step aside so that the teacher can more easily assist. In actual patient care, the patient is not alarmed, the student knows the contract with the teacher will be honoured and the situation is retrieved.

Giving feedback and receiving feedback leads to exploring one's performance and is a critical set of skills for nursing practice. The clinical teacher can introduce these skills into student's practice in the lab.

1. *Planning for intervention for correction:*
   (a) determining criteria and standards of practice to be met;
   (b) clarifying expectations of individual performance;
   (c) providing encouragement through informed support;

   (d) negotiating a contract for intervening in the student's practice.
2. *Giving feedback to students on practical performance*:
   (a) Form a comfortable, open and relaxed relationship in which feedback can be given and received.
   (b) Provide informed comment on performance.
   (c) Give comment immediately after performance.
   (d) Phrase comment in concrete, behavioural terms.
   (e) Choose specific, actual performances for comment.
   (f) Provide written comments on improvement and areas to be improved.
   (g) Give encouragement.
   (h) Ask for feedback on own performance of intervening and giving feedback.

Problem 4. Applying theory to practice

Activity:
Clinical teachers often claim that students find difficulty in making links between their theoretical programme and the actual problems of patients or clients. What are some of the ways you have used to assist your students? After one of your teaching sessions debrief to a colleague on your teaching method and ask her/him to comment.

Feedback:
You may have used problem-solving as an approach which helps students to establish the relevance of and develop associations among several areas of the theoretical programme. If so, you have probably found that problem-solving can be used to integrate basic science and clinical science content in both classroom and clinical sessions. Another approach you may have used is 'learning by active exploration'. In other words, encouraging students to challenge and explore in depth what is being learned. Through this method students can be led to see relationships among separate groups of information and between sequences of learning. Students can be helped to use theory in application to a clinical problem through first learning to integrate the knowledge they have acquired.

What skills can the clinical teacher use in the lab to assist students to apply theory to practice? Learning in the lab can be structured so that students, working together, can assemble material from their theoretical programme in such a way that the relevance of the information for clinical problems is grasped. Take the problem of caring for patients with infectious diseases. The students have had the following relevant subjects in the theoretical programme: physiology, microbiology, social and behavioural sciences, nursing science and human growth and development. The task for the students is to practise ways of applying material from their programme to patients with infectious diseases, such as Hepatitis B.

The teacher can assist students in the following ways.

1. *Encouraging students to identify concepts*: suggest that students rephrase concepts in their own words (to aid conceptualization and to better see the possible ways concepts can be linked).
2. *Assisting them to foster links between the concepts*:
   (a) request students to find ways to order or categorize the concepts;
   (b) encourage them to build a concept map to show how the concepts are linked to form principles.
3. *Promote the exploration of principles*: reward students' initiative in naming principles, using their own words.
4. *Question ways in which the principles can be applied to practice*: provide lab exercises so that students can show how the principles can be directly applied to practice.

Problem 5. Closing the learning/practice gap

This problem is concerned with 'reality shock' experienced by graduates and described by Kramer (1974). Kramer was concerned that the theoretical programme gave students an unrealistic conception of what it was like to be a professional nurse. In Kramer's estimation the gap between the programme and the practice was too large, not only in time, but in language, ideology and patterns of practice, to name a few aspects. Now that programmes in the 1980s and 1990s strive to place students in clinical settings early in the programme so that both theory and practice are experienced contemporaneously, the shock of reality for the graduate may not be such a problem.

In clinical teaching the problem we identified during the clinical teaching project is different. There is still 'shock', but the gap is between one area of clinical practice and another, usually very different, area for which the student is not so well prepared. Specifically, the gap is between what students' experience in clinical practice in the institution and what is expected of them in community care settings. When community experience is left until the later years or months of the programme the gap is very wide indeed because of the overlay of the institutional (hospital) experience which many students perceive to be the approach for all occasions.

Activity:
If you are a clinical teacher in acute care you may never have been on a home visit with one of your students. It would be an interesting project to do so and then together make a list of the different approaches which the student is expected to use in hospital and in the patient's home.

Feedback:
Your reaction to this activity may very well be that it is the responsibility of teachers in community health nursing to identify the learning/practice gap and to advise on how it can be prevented or reduced. However, in the lab, there are frequent opportunities for clinical teachers, whatever their area of specialty, to remind students that much more frequently than in the past, patients or clients are cared for in their own homes. In the simulated lab described earlier (p. 52) the lounge, bedroom and bathroom of a suburban house, as well as the simulated hospital room, enables lab exercises which ask students to change their practice according to the setting. As desirable as that may be it is not sufficient to overcome the learning/practice gap. There needs to be another dimension built into lab teaching which ensures that when any clinical condition and its associated procedures is dealt with the student is prompted by the clinical teacher to suggest how the client will be nursed at home as well as in the familiar hospital room. The overlay of the hospital culture is sufficiently strong to mould students' practice style, role and interactive behaviour as to require deliberate attempts by the clinical teacher to redress the balance.

Competence in clinical skills is only one component of practice whether patients or clients are in hospital or at home. Students also face the complexities that sub-cultures, life-styles and values different from their own, bring to an interaction. Each new encounter, outside the security and familiarity of the hospital structure, brings uncertainty for the student. How can the clinical teacher train for uncertainty?

Structured lab exercises with simulated patients provide ambiguity and challenge students' ability to meet a variety of environments and encourages sensitivity to socio-cultural influences. Role play could also present uncertainty and ambiguity in an hypothetical situation that moves as all players in the scene interact. On the other hand, simulated clients are preferred in training for uncertainty as they would be selected and instructed to represent as closely as possible a real situation in which the student would be required to interact and perform clinical skills.

A number of clinical teaching skills are involved.

1. *Structuring lab exercises*:
   (a) Develop a range of written problems focused on ambiguous, uncertain and unknown situations and outcomes.
   (b) Allow time for processing students' feedback.
   (c) Anticipate students' frustration and provide support.
2. *Providing simulated experiences*:
   (a) Select 'simulated client' wisely.
   (b) Prepare representations of client's environment to give possible context.
   (c) Prepare students by engaging them in preparing ground rules for their activities during the simulation, e.g. notion of 'time-out' and so on.
   (d) Provide for debriefing of participants.
3. *Fostering enquiry into the meaning of the experience*:
   (a) Take time to allow for reflection on the meaning of experiences in the lab.
   (b) Prepare questions to stimulate students' responses and to guide their reflection or, alternatively, allow time for solo reflection then sharing in small groups.
4. *Encouraging students' independence*: prompt students to identify their abilities in
   (a) managing the frustrations during the lab exercises;
   (b) depending on resources other than the teacher's assistance;
   (c) realistic self-appraisal.

It must be said that this problem is related closely to curriculum structure and organization. In programmes where early emphasis is given to nursing roles in primary health care students are aware of the uncertain roles and ambiguous situations of the work of community health nurses. Some programmes are designed to commence student practicum programmes in community settings. The aim is that students will then bring to the hospital setting an understanding of the differences and complexities in some clients' and their families' home and community environments.

3.10 INCREASING MOTIVATION FOR LEARNING IN THE LAB

Activity:
One of the teachers comes to you, as lab co-ordinator, with a problem which has surprised him. The students told him they are bored in the lab. He asks you to help by observing his lab classes. Design an observation schedule for a series of labs so that you can give feedback on his method of motivating his students.

Feedback:
You could construct a sociogram of the interaction in the lab to show teacher–students and student–student communication. This would be an effective, factual way for the lab teacher to grasp whether students are passive while he is instructing, and whether there is a variety of directions of communication so that most of the students are involved. For example, Figure 3.5 shows clearly how the communication flowed in a 'teacher-centred' demonstration, and the number of students involved in a 'student-centred' lab demonstration.

It will be obvious to the lab teacher that there are several strategies which he could use to improve the students' involvement. Separating the cluster of students at the end of the demonstration table or

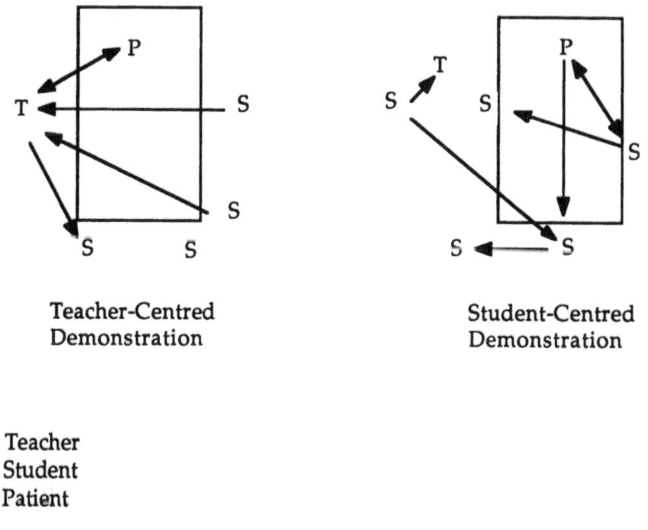

Figure 3.5 Communication in lab-based learning groups.

bed will enable him to have eye-to-eye communication and will remind him to address more of the group with questions, or invite questions from several students in turn. Direct involvement of students in the demonstration has several advantages: involvement of their peers is interesting to the rest of the group; the expectation of being called upon next encourages students to follow closely and to anticipate the next stage of the demonstration; in turn, each student takes a position around the demonstration so that they can be prepared for discussion with the teacher, or with one another.

On another occasion you could take note of the kind of questions the teacher used. A recording could be made of the number of 'closed' (yes/no) questions, or open-ended questions asking for more than simple recall of information and for answers in the student's own words showing understanding of information. The kinds of questions asking students to explore, analyse, discriminate among aspects of a problem, and to trace the steps in their own thinking could also be recorded. In addition, the type of questions the students asked could be detailed as a record of the students' interest and depth of curiosity.

At another lab you could use a schedule of motivating skills and observe whether the lab teacher used the skills, how many times and with what variety they were employed (Table 3.1). The italic headings in the schedule above were adapted from Keller's four major dimensions of motivation from his motivational design model and his explanation of each dimension is as follows:

> interest, which refers to whether the learner's curiosity is aroused and whether this arousal is sustained appropriately over time;
>
> relevance, which refers to whether the learner perceives the instruction to satisfy personal needs or to help achieve personal goals;
>
> expectancy, which refers to the learner's perceived likelihood of success and the extent to which he or she perceives success as being under his or her control;
>
> satisfaction, which refers to the learner's intrinsic motivations and his or her reactions to extrinsic rewards (Keller, 1983, p. 385).

Some helpful hints on motivating students are also given by Salisbury *et al.* (1985). New teachers often prefer to use fairly traditional methods of teaching in the lab because they are unsure that they

Skill	*How used*	*How often*
Gaining attention		
Displaying interest in the topic		
Arousing curiosity		
Providing activity		
Using humour		
Making the demonstration relevant		
Drawing on students' interests and past experiences		
Challenging their possible achievement		
Including ways students can feel personally involved and rewarded		
Building expectancy		
Building confidence		
Emphasizing positive expectancies		
Making criteria for successful performance clear		
Increasing opportunities for experiencing success		
Facilitating satisfaction		
Rewarding interesting practice performance		
Provide unexpected rewards		

Table 3.1 Skill schedule: motivation

will 'cover' all the material required to prepare students for clinical practice if they introduce innovative methods. However, unless students are motivated to become involved, the teacher's well-intentioned efforts could be less than effective and the students' progress in learning and practice may be disappointing.

How can the teacher use attention, interest and curiosity in the lab?

Gaining the attention of students is sometimes difficult if the skill to be learned appears to be mundane. Demonstrations can often be boring if students are not included actively or their attention has not been grasped. Providing variation in the overall style of the demonstration or presentation such that the style changes from active to passive, fast to slow, or humorous to serious is often effective.

Attention occurs when something unexpected happens in the student's environment, or when there is a gap between what a student knows and what he/she sees is desirable to know. Presenting a humorous, puzzling or curious yet credible example of a problem in a practice situation can gain attention. For example, an event from the teacher's own experience, told graphically. 'How do you think I solved it; what do you think I did?'

Attention is actually a complex perceptual sensory-level reaction (Reigeluth, 1983, p. 399). Teachers often use curiosity to gain attention and to maintain selective attention by doing something startling at the beginning or later during a presentation. This strategy is effective but usually captures attention only momentarily. The difficulty of using loud noises, or dropping trays, or other attention-getting distractions in the lab is that the clinical teacher is also trying to model a smooth, professional performance. A more effective attention-getting device is to arrange to have a volunteer from the community (for example a personality likely to raise the interest and curiosity of the student group) intrude just at the beginning of a demonstration and agree to act as the 'patient' during the demonstration.

Attention through information-seeking and problem-solving is more sustained and builds its own sequential steps. In programmes where problem-solving is the preferred approach to learning appropriate time is made available for students to work on problems linking the practice in the lab with an actual patient or client. The important point is to exploit students' curiosity by allowing them to explore, manipulate and act on their environment.

In any lab, activity in a challenging, yet safe situation is motivating so long as the challenge is neither too difficult, nor too simple. For example: ask students to role play a mother and child and nurse in a clinic – the child (student) has to receive an injection – how would the child (student) want this to happen? How would the nurse give the injection?

How can the clinical teacher make the lab relevant to students' needs?

To sustain motivation, students must perceive that the skill is relevant not only to their clinical practice but also to their own personal needs. Usually there is at least one student in the group who knows or has heard of the particular condition being discussed, or has personal experience of the intervention being demonstrated. Draw upon the student's interests and past experiences in relation to the skill to be practised. Open the possibility for students to suggest alternative methods of practice to accomplish the same goal.

Students' need for achievement can be stimulated by enabling them to practise under conditions of challenge so that they can achieve standards of excellence. Individual contracting, or group contracting with specified criteria for success and moderate risk can be motivating. Be clear about how the practice relates to the student's future activities. Achieving the initial immediate goals will be more motivating when they are perceived to be steps toward accomplishing a future more desired goal (Salisbury *et al.*, 1985).

The need for affiliation, Maslow (1954) suggests, is important to be met before people will engage in activities which could challenge their self-esteem. Allay students' fear of rejection by creating opportunities for establishing trust between teacher and student and among group members. Introduce co-operative activities (such as pairs or partners) rather than competition between individuals in the performance of lab tasks.

Students' expectancy of success can be nurtured in the lab. What can the clinical teacher do to increase their confidence? Make sure that the expected performance and the criteria for successful performance are stated clearly. Also 'increase the expectancy of success by increasing experience with success' (Reigeluth, 1983, p. 418). It is the increase in the expectancy of success which will lead to improved confidence. While it is true that reinforcement of correct performance is motivational, the response a person makes is dependent on the continued attraction of the reinforcer. On the other hand, the expectancy of success is more cognitive than behavioural. Thinking that one will be successful, accompanied by previous successful performance, appears to be the optimal combination.

The emphasis on positive expectancies implies that the tasks must not be trivial or too easy, and must be similar to those the student will be required to perform in the clinical setting. In brief:

1. Begin a practice session with the more easily attainable skills.
2. Present the practice steps in identifiable units.
3. Give feedback that supports student ability and effort.
4. Redesign practice activities which frequently cause failure.

Techniques that offer personal control over success are useful in improving students' confidence. Individual contracting, including the criteria for evaluation is an example. In lab work, which extends into clinical practice, individual contracts enable students to indicate exactly what it is they want to achieve, in both lab and clinical.

Some students have developed a 'learned helplessness' attitude towards some aspects of lab and clinical work. They will work on easy lab problems but will ease off when the challenges are more difficult. There seems to be little understanding of the connection between persistence and ability in achieving success. To some extent the clinical teacher, unintentionally, can contribute to 'learned helplessness' by protecting the student from challenges in a belief that support is what the student needs most. A judicious choice of graded problems in an easy-to-difficult sequence in an atmosphere of support and challenge can motivate students to succeed. It is important to follow each successful outcome by comments to indicate that persistence, effort and trying are as important as ability (Salisbury *et al.*, 1985).

The fourth component of Keller's (1983) major dimensions of motivation is satisfaction. How can learner satisfaction be gained in the lab? To gain satisfaction from performance, students need to feel that the rewards gained from an activity are in tune with their expectations. It is important to provide opportunities for practice of a newly acquired skill in the clinical setting as soon as possible. Satisfaction is also attained by students when they are recognized for their performance. For example, suggest to those who have mastered a skill that they could help others to practise the skill.

Satisfaction is often gained through the performance of intrinsically interesting practice. The teacher can give unexpected rewards for this performance as it is additional to the satisfaction from the experience itself. On the other hand, when practice is sometimes unavoidably predictable and mundane, satisfaction can be gained when the teacher gives fair, anticipated rewards (Salisbury *et al.*, 1985).

3.11 REACTIONS OF LEARNERS IN THE LAB

Activity:
Your students have asked you to meet with them to discuss the proposed changes in the laboratory sessions. They also want to put to the faculty their comments on learning in the laboratory. Can you anticipate their comments? What will be the most likely points that facilitate, or alternatively, hinder their learning in the lab?

Feedback:
Informal talks with students often reveal some basic attitudes towards their learning. When these attitudes are shared by the group rather than being a personal view by one or two individual students, the faculty needs to know in the students' own words what helps them and what hinders them in laboratory learning. Formal written evaluations by students are also sources of valuable information. Face-to-face discussion gives opportunities for probing more deeply to gain more precise feedback about their progress in learning to nurse. To what extent have you heard the following comments from your students?

It helps me when:

1. we can watch someone do something and then do it ourselves;
2. I am allowed to learn by my own initiative;
3. I am working by myself without much active interference;
4. I am left to my own resources without being over-protected;
5. I am working alone but knowing there is help if I need it;
6. there is always a tutor available to refer to;
7. I have plenty of practice even if it means repetition of a particular skill;
8. I get feedback as the task is being done, not later;
9. I can accept calm positive correction of specific errors;
10. my mistakes are pointed out, so that there is not a habit of doing things half right;
11. I get really useful feedback, but I do not want pressure to be always right – I can learn best by my own mistakes in the lab, and by the mistakes of others too;
12. we have practice in the duties we are supposed to perform as well as each of the tasks;
13. I am encouraged to ask questions;
14. I have adequate practical sessions at college;
15. I can have nursing practicals the afternoon before the clinical;
16. we practise on each other as it helps me to understand how it would feel to be the patient;
17. I am encouraged to try new situations;
18. when there is time for discovery – time on my own, with feedback with sufficient explanation to understand where I could improve;
19. when the teacher is involved as a colleague;
20. there's no time-wasting; no tutorials (*sic*); mostly practice and feedback.

Activity:
How do these students see the teacher's role in the lab? How do you see your role? Identifying your role as a teacher in the lab is one way of summarizing the major issues raised by this chapter. Compare your answers with the feedback below.

3.12 THE ROLE OF THE CLINICAL TEACHER IN THE LAB

Feedback:
The random comments above from a group of first-year nursing students leave no doubt that lab sessions are crucial in their preparation for clinical practice and the teacher's role can help or hinder their learning. In summary the roles suggested by the students' comments are:

1. *Colleague*, involved, interested, giving honest feedback, but not being over-protective, accepts each student and gives encouragement knowing that judgement of performance will come not from one poor performance but from the full range of abilities, attitudes and performances as a whole.
2. *Facilitator*, recognizing when students want to be 'left to their own resources' but not necessarily alone; being available but not intrusive; being sensitive to when they need encouragement and when 'correction of specific errors' is required to prevent 'doing things half right'; allowing students to learn by their own mistakes; and above all, it seems, building confidence.
3. *Expert clinician*, credible, with the authority that comes with 'knowing how and why' and with the skills of including students in demonstrations of complex as well as simple and/or mundane clinical simulations.
4. *Manager and co-ordinator*, designing interesting exercises, having resources available, making sure that time is not wasted and that practice sessions are timed as closely as possible before clinical practice sessions.
5. *Challenger*, introducing new situations to test individual ability, extending individual students intellectually and practically, expecting high standards.
6. *Helper*, relieving the pressure for students to be right every time; making realistic allowances for individual fatigue, anxieties and lapses in knowledge or performance.

You may agree that your role in the lab includes all of the above dimensions but with the following additional roles:

7. *Assessor*, making observations of direct performance in the lab and making judgements according to explicit expectations, standards and criteria, known well in advance of assessments and applying equally to each student, engendering trust, fairness and reliability.
8. *Researcher*, preparing students to apply theory to practice, and finding ways to derive theory from practice, building co-operative and collaborative relationships with students, stimulating enquiry, encouraging discovery.

4

The briefing: preparing students for clinical practice

4.1 INTRODUCTION

The briefing or pre-conference session has a special place in the clinical learning cycle (Figure 4.1). Its links with debriefing after clinical practice highlight the cyclical nature of clinical teaching. Whilst the lab is important in enabling students to master sets of clinical skills in a low-risk environment, the briefing–clinical practice–debriefing cycle concentrates on the students' clinical assignments in the real world of clinical/community practice. Each of the three stages is distinct and well-defined demanding special skills of the clinical teacher and students. At the same time, each stage is linked to the others; the clinical teacher and students continue through the cycle in a gradual spiral to mirror the students' progression from stage to stage.

Students are usually impatient to get into clinical practice. For them, it is the pinnacle, the reason they are learning to nurse. Its value depends on the strength of their preparation for practice and the analysis after the experience. In the lab students practised in a simulated environment, sometimes with simulated clients. When they move on to the 'real thing' they are expected to be equipped with appropriate technical skills and some understanding of the complexities of the context in which they will use their skills. Not surprisingly, they have concerns about their lack of experience of practice and their knowledge of the clients they will nurse during the clinical assignments they are given.

How can the clinical teacher assist students to prepare for clinical assignments? What is the purpose of the briefing or pre-conference session? Is a briefing session always necessary, always possible?

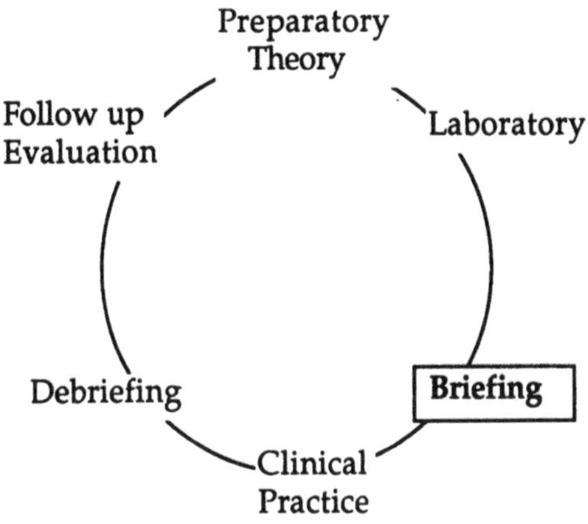

Figure 4.1 Clinical learning cycle: briefing.

Ideally, how many students can be involved in a briefing session? What skills does the clinical teacher need to ensure an effective briefing session? Where should the briefing session be held? How long should it take? What has been the experience of clinical teachers in conducting briefing sessions?

This chapter aims to address these questions and to draw on the experiences of clinical teachers in their attempts to design and conduct effective briefing or pre-conference sessions. By the end of this chapter you will have reviewed the purposes of the briefing session in your own programme, assessed its value for preparing your students for clinical practice and identified the clinical teaching skills necessary for effective briefing sessions.

4.2 ARE BRIEFING SESSIONS NECESSARY?

The term 'briefing' is usually associated with short, precise directions before a mission or exercise, e.g. armed forces task force or civilian security measures. As was noted in Chapter 2, the practice has an established place in clinical supervision in teacher education (Goldhammer, 1969; Turney *et al.*, 1982; Smyth, 1986) and in professional education generally (Boud *et al.*, 1985). Nursing education programmes have adapted it as a 'pre-conference' before clinical practice (Matheney, 1969) and we will now consider its relevance for clinical teaching.

Activity:
Your group of eight clinical students are attending your theoretical module and are beginning its clinical component. They have had an orientation to the ward, and have met the staff and the clients. Are briefing sessions really necessary for these students? Jot down your reasons if you believe they are.

Feedback:
Your reasons for taking the time and effort to conduct briefing sessions may be related to the structure and requirements of your programme, but it is important that you have a clear aim in mind which will direct the way you plan and conduct the session.

Your students are part of a large class (perhaps between 100 and 200) attending your module. They have worked in lab session (in groups of, say, 20–30) and you may know some of this small briefing group already. Is the lab not enough preparation for your students? You will be with them during their clinical assignment where you will have opportunities for clarification, instruction and facilitation. Would not the time be better spent in the clinical setting with these students who are all keen to get started?

One of the first to write on pre-conference (or briefing) discussions in nursing education, Matheney (1969) notes that they were developed first in associate degree nursing programmes in the USA and were designed with a definite purpose, structure and direction. Her approach has stood the test of time but inevitably modifications and adaptations have appeared (DiRienzo, 1983). In re-examining clinical teaching Infante (1985) suggests that the briefing session can be de-emphasized, or even omitted, if the college lab has been effective in preparing students for the clinical experience. In fact briefing (or pre-conference) is seldom mentioned in detail in recent nursing literature with the exception of Carpenito and Duespohl (1985) and Reilly and Oermann (1985) who include pre-conferences within a short section on conferencing.

What then is the importance of briefing sessions?

In recent years the preparation of students for clinical practice has become important as nurse education has moved into mainstream higher education. No longer is exposure to, or time spent in, a clinical area considered to be sufficient preparation for the care of clients. The clinical teacher's responsibilities are not limited to a supervisory role while students carry out a clinical assignment, but include preparation of students so that maximum benefit is gained from the clinical experience.

We have taken the view in the clinical learning cycle that the purposes of the lab (see Chapter 3) are related to students' learning to apply from the theoretical programme those key concepts which are relevant to many skills and many situations and not a particular context or patient. The major purpose of the briefing session is its focus on the *particular patient* who is the subject of the student's assignment and on preparing students for that particular clinical episode. This means addressing not only their practical preparation, but also their readiness and concerns.

If you accept the view that reflection and debriefing are important aspects of learning from experience you will also see the briefing session as a necessary component in preparing for reflective learning. The sequential nature of clinical teaching, from theoretical programme, to lab, briefing, clinical practice and debriefing is in direct contrast to conventional clinical teaching. The latter, by force of circumstance jumped directly from lecture hall to teaching skills at the bedside. Patient, student and teacher were all ill-prepared.

You may have other reasons for considering briefing sessions are necessary apart from your direct clinical teaching/learning responsibilities. Some of your reasons may be concerned with clinical issues related to your area of speciality and with the opportunity to work through students' questions. Or you may be especially interested or engaged in clinical research, which again, can be discussed with students.

Consider again the reasons you wrote down for conducting briefing sessions. Is your personal, educational and professional interest sufficient to motivate your students? DiRienzo (1983) reports that students lapsed into a 'passive recipient role' in her sessions, requiring later remedial briefing in the clinical setting. Will your motivation urge you to create a briefing session which will involve students actively and creatively?

4.3 PURPOSES OF THE BRIEFING SESSION

Apart from your own reasons about the necessity of briefing sessions, your school or faculty will have defined the purposes of briefing sessions in your programme. They may be available as a written list. Alternatively, they may simply be an unwritten common understanding. Whatever form the briefing takes, its major purpose is usually understood to be 'preparation of students for clinical practice'. The breadth of that statement leaves new clinical teachers in some difficulty. Mitchell and Krainovich (1982) admit uncertainties in their early experiences and found echoes of themselves in new faculty members. When DiRienzo (1983) reviewed the purposes of the pre-conference she found them to be far more encompassing than she had realized.

In Matheney's (1969) terms the purposes were '(1) to provide direction for learning for the day; (2) to set groundwork for analysis of the experience; (3) to recognize the scope and limitations of the nurse's role; and (4) to reinforce "process" learning, for example, problem-solving, application of knowledge, and use of judgment' (p. 286). These purposes continue to be important, and other purposes have been added during the ensuing 20 years to reflect the changing view of the power and impact of experience in clinical practice.

But what is it, exactly, that you are preparing your students for in clinical? How will you identify what your briefing sessions are aiming to do, beyond the broad 'preparing students for clinical practice?'

Activity:
Imagine that you have accepted that the purposes for the briefing sessions in your current module are to prepare students

1. for learning in the clinical setting;
2. for the activities of a clinical assignment;
3. for a clinical experience.

Write objectives for a briefing session based on each purpose in terms of what you want the students to achieve.

Feedback:

Preparing students for learning in the clinical setting

If this is the first briefing session in your module your main objectives may include your aim that students should know what the briefing session is about and that they should assist in determining the focus of the session. The briefing session is an ideal opportunity for making clear the expectations and limitations of the students' performance.

Based on the well-documented evidence of students' anxiety and stress in new clinical settings (Turkoski, 1987; Pagana, 1988; Dennis, 1989; Kleehammer *et al.*, 1990) your objectives may include your intention to create a low-risk, comfortable, non-judgemental atmosphere and to assist students to identify their concerns so that you may find ways to reduce their stress and increase their confidence. Reducing the stress of students unfamiliar with the area, the staff and the clients, is essential before students are ready for clinical practice.

Although you may know some (or all) of the students it is better to assume that one of the major purposes of this first briefing session is for you and the students to know each other better and to help the students to feel at ease by making the environment as physically and emotionally comfortable as possible. This is especially important if you wish the students to regard you and each other as colleagues in their clinical assignments. Dennis (1989) in an investigation of clinical students' support networks, discovered that students more often sought support from their peers than from the clinical teacher. What implications does this have for the purposes of the briefing session? It could mean that identifying students' concerns is of major importance. Because students usually want to appear in a good light they may be reluctant to voice their concerns in front of the teacher. Objectives related to sensitive questioning and use of peer support in the group can assist you in uncovering the major areas of concern.

The uncertainty of clinical demands is likely to be a cause of anxiety; your objectives might therefore include contracting to support a student for certain aspects of the experience. Knowledge that the student will not be alone and vulnerable will provide reassurance. When confidence is restored you may then both agree to end the contract for that episode. Since you will be with these students during their clinical assignments you may wish to include objectives focusing on establishing a colleague relationship with students so that your roles are made explicit.

While a certain degree of direction may be necessary, your objectives may also deal with assisting students to identify their learning needs in relation to the skills they already possess and those they wish to master. The programme may already specify what students are to learn as well as what they are to do in the clinical assignment e.g. learning how to improve their interaction skills with patients, by noting in a journal what they consider to be the characteristics of their effective and/or ineffective interactions (learning how to learn), as well as interviewing a patient to make a health status assessment (the learning task). In addition, students often have learning needs related to their personal growth. Even in the first briefing your objectives may include an intention to give students permission and power to explore their own needs and potential for personal and professional growth, by simple invitations such as 'Let me know what you would like to work on in the area of ___ and how you would like me to work with you'. You might want to include in your objectives a somewhat more formal strategy of assisting students to design a contract to meet a particular need they have expressed. If you intend furthering your students' self-directive learning needs, you may also wish to include an objective in those terms.

Clinical learning is a complex activity requiring a synthesis of content from various fields, a familiarity with the client's problems, and practice in how to use problem-solving to assist application and transfer of knowledge and skills in the resolution of clients' problems. Your objectives for the briefing session may include the intention to engender a problem-solving group process in the briefing session which becomes the primary teaching/learning strategy of each briefing session and, in turn, will become the strategy students will use in learning in the clinical setting.

Preparing students for the activities of a clinical assignment

The preparatory task has two stages. First, selection of the clinical assignment and secondly, preparation of the students.

Selection of the clinical assignment. Depending on your students' level of learning, and the objectives of the programme, the clinical assignment may be care of a patient or a group of patients. Early in the programme, however, the assignment is more likely to be a graduated, less complex assignment to give experience in development of skills, e.g. taking vital signs and/or interacting with patients. (The selection of clinical assignments and experiences will be dealt with in more detail in Chapter 5).

Interestingly, McCoin and Jenkins (1988) outline five ways of selecting clinical assignments depending on the degree of involvement of the clinical teacher, the student and the staff of the facility. The degree of involvement students have, or have not, had in the selection of clients and assignments will be influential in their preparation for the assignment. They may, or may not, have prior knowledge of the clients and the relevant background information. Your principal objective in preparing students will, therefore, reflect your intention to ascertain the readiness of students for the assignment. The importance of affirming the students' relevant background knowledge, requisite skills and the problems which might arise, cannot be over-stated in relation to the students' safety to practise and self-confidence during the assignment.

Preparation of the student for the assignment. The major question the clinical teacher can prompt the students to ask is 'why do I have this particular assignment and what will I learn from it?' One way of ensuring that students are clear about the nature of the assignment is to assist them to develop skills in assessing the clinical objectives they have been given (e.g. for specificity, clarity, feasibility and relevance to their stage of learning and practice) or in developing their own clinical objectives. This may lead into preparing students to check their nursing care plans for the assignment, identifying possible problems and rehearsing selected techniques of practice.

Andersen (1990b) offers advice on preparing students for the assignment and suggests that the clinical teacher needs to include objectives that are framed to

> allow the learner to *develop a sense of responsibility by being responsible*; the ability to initiate, and manage and evaluate wisely by "rehearsing" these skills; the ability to engage continuously in a meaningful learning process by carrying out the learning themselves (p. 5).

Assisting students to link their current assignment with previous experiences or assignments may be framed in an objective which prepares them to see a progressive increase in their knowledge, understanding and skills. Depending on the stage of students in the programme you may also include in your objectives an intention that students progress in learning to apply theory to practice and/or to develop skills in uncovering theory from practice. This would involve a determination, over the period of the clinical module, of the students' understanding of theory and their ability to apply it and underscores the advantages of teaching an integrated theory and clinical module.

Preparing for experience

What is the experience you are intending students should have and how will you prepare them for it? In the past, clinical experience was regarded as time spent in a clinical area, or the range of areas of practice covered during the programme or the skills developed by the 'experienced' practitioner. It is clear that clinical experience is much more than that. To Benner and Wrubel, (1982b) it means 'living through actual situations in such a way that it informs the practitioner's perceptions and understanding of all subsequent situations' (p. 14).

How will you prepare students for that kind of experience? What objectives will you decide for this component of the briefing session? Dewey (1938) asked a similar question of educational experience: 'What is the true meaning of preparation in the educational scheme?' (p. 49) and cautioned that it is a fallacy to think that 'a person learns only the particular thing he is studying at the time' (p. 48). Dewey believed that preparation for experience 'means that a person, young or old, gets out of his present experience all that there is in it for him at the time in which he has it' and 'this means that attentive care must be devoted to the conditions which give each present experience a worthwhile meaning' (p. 49) rather than 'using the present simply to get ready for the future' (p. 49).

If we interpret Dewey's explanation to mean that the clinical assignment of students is not the only thing students are learning we must consider the influence of the 'complex, unstable, uncertain and conflictual worlds of practice' (Schon, 1988, p. 11) on the students' experience. Preparation for experience offers an important challenge that clinical teachers have often not fully recognized. Certainly, the debriefing session provides opportunities for deriving meaning from the experience, but the quality of the preparation before the experience potentially determines the effectiveness of the later reflection and exploration.

Schon believes that reflection begins much earlier than after the experience and it is, in fact, reflection-in-action which gives meaning to the experience. Surprising events or situations are not uncommon in clinical practice. When this happens Schon explains that 'We consider both the unexpected event and the knowing-in-action that led up to it, asking ourselves, as it were, "What is it?" and at the same time, "How have I been thinking about it?"' (p. 28). In so doing we are rethinking, responding and reacting on-the-spot.

In this sense students become independent learners as they are learning to interpret what is happening during their experience. No one else can have this experience for them; no one else can know what the experience means for them at the time (Boud *et al.*, 1985). In fact, Schon (1988) points out that 'reflection-in-action is a process we can deliver without being able to say what we are doing' (p. 31).

What difference does this make to the way the clinical teacher prepares students for learning in the clinical setting and for the activities of the clinical assignment? There are elements of technical (craft-like) and practical (process) training (Carr and Kemmis, 1986) woven into those components. Certainly, during the experience, students are learning by doing, involving rules, facts and procedures, and practising in a complex, changing environment of social and political relationships. Moreover, according to Schon (1988), when students 'sometimes make new sense of uncertain, unique or conflicted situations of practice' they are freeing themselves in their thinking to go beyond the boundaries of technical practice to question their previously accepted styles of thinking and practice. Carr and Kemmis point to 'critical self-reflection' as a result of the systematic examination which is sometimes possible in the practice situation.

> To the extent that it is possible, (the student) plans thoughtfully, acts deliberately, observes the consequences of actions systematically, and reflects critically on the situational constraints and practical potential of the strategic action being considered (Carr and Kemmis, 1986, p. 40).

If that is what 'the experience' engenders, Schon urges that 'instructors function more as coaches than as teachers' (p. 20). Smyth (1984) describes a similar coaching role in teacher education. Through a genuine sharing relationship, 'The aim is to uncover the (student's) intentions and see how these are expected to be translated into practice' (p. 7). The student's 'intentions' for the experience may be a private world which remains closed to the clinical teacher. Included in your objectives may be the aim to share with students your intentions for your experience and so relate as a 'coach', demonstrating, inviting joint experimentation and building relationships (Schon, 1988). Unique, colleague relationships with individual students could result, as part of both the briefing and the clinical practice sessions. In fact, it is important to remember that your coaching extends into the clinical practice session to follow; your objectives may then include developing your assessment of what individual students understand about the potential of the experience, what difficulties they may have and what they already know how to do.

4.4 PREPARING FOR THE BRIEFING SESSION

Activity:
Students and clinical teacher have responsibilities to come to the briefing session well prepared. What are your expectations for stu-

dents preparedness for a briefing session? What preparation will you have made?

Make two lists, one for students, one for yourself. Try to line up the lists to see if they correspond in order to achieve an effective briefing session.

Feedback:
It is possible that students know what is expected of them in preparing for a briefing session since that may be specified in guidelines, or in course handbooks. Your module, however, may have different or additional requirements which need to be made clear to students, for example, your policy on students who are obviously unprepared for the clinical assignment. Depending on the individual student's circumstances and/or reason for unpreparedness, will the student be permitted to practise on that day, or altenatively, should she/he be given an assignment more appropriate to the knowledge, ability or personal approach of the student?

Table 4.1 is an outline of basic activities for preparing for a module of clinical teaching and learning. What similarities and differences are there between this list and the one you made? Which of these activities would you omit, or what additional points would you want to include? Is the schedule of preparation realistic for your situation? Given the importance of preparing students for clinical practice, what constraints (or facilitators) are operating to influence your proposal? How will you amend your preparation to take account of the demands of the physical situation, availability of a suitable room, access to suitable clinical assignments, previous experience of students, your own familiarity with the clinical setting and your clinical competence, and lastly your relationship with the clinical staff of the area?

4.5 PLANNING A PROGRAMME OF BRIEFING SESSIONS

This section includes the following:

1. setting objectives;
2. identifying student outcomes;
3. selecting teaching/learning strategies;
4. sequencing the sessions;
5. organizing the session.

Depending on your knowledge of the students, their level in the programme and the nature of the clinical setting, you will need to

Teacher	*Student*
Create a clinical teaching programme into which this briefing will fit	
Consider the student group, level, experience and characteristics	Revise material from module to prepare for clinical briefing
Check that students have necessary information of time, place and programme. Schedule briefing immediately prior to clinical practice session	Read resource materials; check-out place and time
Consider any influences on students' readiness to learn, e.g. time of day, fatigue, impending exams, assignments	Alert clinical teacher to any overlaps in exams, programme, schedules, etc. well before the day. Have an early night
Realize the nature of students' anxieties in clinical settings and prepare strategies to reduce stress	
Develop a written plan of the sessions with suggested objectives, focus, teaching learning/methods and timed sequence of events. Include lists of questions for students to be used in finalizing plans for the session. Distribute to students ahead of time. Anticipate students' questions and consider responses	Go over the suggested plan. What are your reactions? Share with a friend What are the surprises, disappointmnts, joys, bonuses? Work through it before the session
Consider what follow-up learning students should be given to prepare for next briefing session	Ask yourself 'what do I want to learn from this clinical module?'
Acquire appropriate resources for small group learning – comfort of room, quiet, easy access to clinical setting	
Choose appropriate clients, seek their permission, give explanation and seek co-operation	Go with clinical teacher to choose clients or visit later (within limits of time and comfort of client)
Check ward routine and any possibility that client care activity will affect availability	
Elicit co-operation of ward staff	

Table 4.1 Preparing for the briefing session

make decisions about the sequence, structure and direction of the briefing session. If you are to spend the next few weeks with these students you might consider a progressive plan of briefing sessions which you could work out with the students. Your instructional design could take into consideration the need to link briefing and debriefing and to discuss with the students their progress in clinical learning.

In Chapter 2 we considered the contribution of experiential learning theorists to clinical learning, and the influence of other approaches such as problem-based, concept-based and competency-based learning on structuring learning experiences. Remember also the recent work on the 'reflective practitioner' and its potential for influencing clinical learning in nursing. Keep these influences in mind as we consider how to plan for and conduct briefing sessions. You may already have extensive experience in briefing your students and you may now wish to try other approaches. For example, structuring briefing in relation to the debriefing session after clinical practice, or using a variation of enquiry techniques. In essence, a briefing session is a small group activity, but sometimes can be one-to-one. Facilitating small group work is dealt with in many general education texts as well as texts for teachers of nursing (Schweer, 1972; de Tornyay, 1982). Although in this text we are concerned with those clinical teaching skills and strategies which are different from, and/or complementary to, the skills of classroom teaching, it is useful to include an example of small group facilitation at this point. The following extract from Ewan and White (1984) addresses the skills of planning a small group session and could be used for clinical learning in small groups.

Activity:
Plan a small group session for a topic that you teach. Pay particular attention to the following:

1. How will you introduce the topic?
2. How will you encourage participation by group members?
3. How will you finish off the discussion or activity?

Feedback:
Needless to say that you should begin your planning by deciding what the objectives of the learning session are. Don't forget that since you are using a small group for the topic you should try to include objectives which make use of the capacity for

practice, interaction and feedback. In other words you should use the small group as an opportunity for attitudes and skill learning as well as the acquisition of knowledge. Since you may not always have complete control over the direction in which students take the discussion you should give careful thought to the *key areas* or *key questions* which you would like to be addressed by the group. If their discussions take them into those areas well and good, if not you can be prepared to judiciously insert probing or leading questions which will bring those key issues to the fore.

Decide on the level of autonomy you wish the group to have and therefore on the level of control you wish to exert over the activities of the group. If you intend to maintain a low profile it will be particularly important for you to provide an introduction to the topic which will allow the students to define its scope and direction without having to guess what you want them to do.

The following suggestions are an incomplete list of strategies you may use for getting the group started and keeping it going.

Starting the group discussion

The way you start the discussion would motivate students to want to talk about the topic or undertake the task.

- Use a case study, film or story to focus students on the topic and help them to see its relevance to the tasks of the nurse.
- Show enthusiasm for the topic and an interest in tackling the problem or procedure yourself.
- Try to choose a problem or task that the students see as important – you might want to involve them in the choice of specific topics or tasks to be undertaken.
- Clearly define the problem or topic to be addressed and the nature of the task confronting the group. Tell them the objectives or enlist their aid in defining or modifying the objectives.

Encouraging group participation

- Arrange seating in such a way that group members can freely talk to each other.
- Try to ensure that group members are prepared for the discussion by notifying them of the topic in advance, prescribing prior activities or prereading assignments.

- Resist the temptation to talk too much and provide all the answers. Given enough time to become comfortable and to think, most group members find that they can contribute usefully to each other's knowledge and skills.
- Be aware of the stages that groups pass through and be prepared to help the group through difficult phases. Ask gently probing questions which focus the discussion and encourage quieter group members to speak.
- Be aware of the various roles that members of the group are assuming, and of the ways in which they participate, and be prepared to help them to learn effective ways to contribute to the discussion or task.

Finishing off the discussion

- Warn students 10 minutes before the end of time so that they can come to some conclusions or closure in their discussion or task.
- Summarise or encourage the students to summarise the discussion and highlight the main points discussed and the main achievements in relation to the objectives.
- Review the work which still needs to be done and set the task for the next meeting.

(Ewan and White, 1984.)

DiRienzo (1983) claims that although nursing faculty consider preclinical conferences are useful, information on how to conduct them effectively is not available and that 'most often they are ritualistically planned for a given amount of time at the beginning of every experience in the clinical lab setting' (p. 84).

To make planning the briefing sessions less a matter of 'ritual' and more likely to meet your objectives it is helpful to specify what you want your students to achieve in the briefing sessions and then to select an appropriate teaching/learning strategy.

Activity:
Look again at the objectives you wrote for your briefing sessions. Each objective can be used to identify the learning you want students to achieve and you can then select a teaching/learning strategy.

Make three columns: in the first list your objectives, the next column is headed expected student outcome and the third teaching learning strategies. Enter a student outcome and a teaching/learning strategy for each objective.

Feedback:
It is possible that the way you have written the objectives contains both what you want the students to achieve and the teaching/learning process. The maxim 'embed the process in the objective' is a helpful reminder of this facility. Table 4.2 shows a few examples. When you have completed the table of objectives, expected student outcomes and teaching/learning strategies you can use it as the basis for the sequence, organization and implementation of the programme of briefing sessions in the module.

Sequencing the briefing sessions

Take a few moments to scan your objectives. Which ones are more important for students at the beginning of the clinical module? You will probably choose to spend the first briefing session on 'getting to know each other', 'identifying students' concerns about the clinical area in general' and allaying their anxiety and reducing their stress. This could be followed by a short clinical exposure (such as a brief interview with clients to obtain background information for a later clinical assignment, or an observation exercise to study the placement of facilities in the ward or clinic). It is important that students

Objective	*Expected student outcome*	*Teaching/learning strategies*
Establish a colleague relationship with students so that the roles of students and teacher are made explicit	Knowledge of role in relationship, and commitment to colleagueship	Role play to identify roles, negotiation of roles, decision making for commitment
Assisting students to identify their learning needs in relation to the skills they already possess and those they wish to master	Personal learning needs recorded in own words, graphs or picture and relevant to their level of learning	'Time-out' exercise with pencil and paper: 'Where am I now? Where do I want to be by the end of this module?'
and so on . . .		
—	—	—

Table 4.2 Examples of objectives for briefing sessions

have direction and a prescribed amount of time for the first short experience. The direction could be in the form of questions to be answered later, a journal entry to record, or a review of the experience to bring to a debriefing session.

The cyclical and developmental nature of students' experiences will direct the sequencing of the remaining briefing sessions. Once students are less anxious, the clinical assignments can be selected to reflect their increased confidence and skills, and more of the briefing time will then be spent on preparation for specific assignments. In turn, the impact of the clinical experience on individual students will need to be addressed, and later in the module the briefing sessions could give more emphasis to preparing students for deeper understanding of their experiences in the clinical setting.

Organizing the briefing sessions

Several factors are important here:

1. Frequency of the sessions – are they each day before every clinical assignment or experience, or at the beginning of a week or a series of experiences?
2. The level of knowledge and skill of your students determines how often briefing sessions are necessary. Other factors are the proximity or remoteness of students' placements and the logistics of meeting together.
3. Time allowed for each session – must it be the same every time, or can you expand or contract it to suit your purposes? Matheney's (1969) sessions took from 20 minutes to one hour for a teacher-led discussion, using the remaining (unspecified) time for setting clinical assignments with students in the clinical setting.
4. The time of day – is it the same time each day, e.g. 7 a.m. before clinical practice? Is it possible to vary the time during the day to capture aspects of practice for which students need to be 'briefed'?
5. Location of the session – there are advantages in obtaining a room adjacent to the clinical setting if possible. As well as reducing travelling time, the proximity to the demands of clinical places the briefing session in a realistic context. The briefing session does not always have to be held in a conference room for the entire time. Moving in and out of clinical to obtain information is a possibility and avoids the tendency to 'decontextualize' the focus of the session. Remembering that physical

comfort is an important condition for learning, keep a watch on the time students spend on their feet in a 'walk-around' briefing or, alternatively, is there a suitable place for your sessions with sufficient seating and room for role play or slide projector or video?

6. The possible involvement of clinical staff to explain and negotiate the programme and liasion about the use of facilities. An interesting variation of the pre- and post-conference suggests a 'three-way-conference where student, teacher and clinical staff are involved, each with a specific role' (Fishel and Johnson, 1981).

4.6 CONDUCTING THE BRIEFING SESSION

Innovations and alternatives

Many clinical teachers have approached the conduct of briefing sessions as a fairly straight-forward educational activity consisting of teacher led discussions of unfamiliar material, small group interaction and student presentations of nursing care plans or clinical assignment activities. This is basic, tried and tested classroom teaching. It is true that briefing usually occurs in an environment similar to a classroom. However, the close proximity and imminent demands of practice mean that briefing is a significant component of clinical practice (in essence, 'looking before leaping'). Moreover, it is a unique opportunity for helping the student to anticipate and eventually to discover what it means to be a nurse. Individual strengths and weaknesses can be identified and faced in a supportive session. Steps can then be initiated, with each student, towards further strengthening and improvement before unrealistic self-assessments by students themselves confirm either their fears of inadequacy or their false sense of their own ability.

In addition, the cyclical nature of clinical teaching suggests that it is worthwhile to consider a method that allows interaction between each stage so that continuity of focus is retained for each student group. This is more important than appears at first. If the clinical teacher believes that the purpose of the clinical programme is to demonstrate to students not only the skills, processes, techniques and attitudes involved in caring, but an approach to practice that can be used whatever the setting or the clinical/community problem, then the preparation for and reflection after clinical practice are ways of practising and are as important as the clinical assignment component. A series of unconnected briefing, clinical practice and debriefing sessions is the antithesis of what is intended by the clinical learning cycle. It is not surprising that 'Innovative approaches to clinical conferences are clearly one of the profession's most pressing concerns' (Skurski, 1985, p. 166).

Activity:
Remember that the briefing session does not stand alone, but is part of a cycle of preparation for clinical practice, followed by experience in clinical practice and later by a debriefing session. The purposes of the briefing session in preparing students for learning, for the clinical assignment and for the experience suggest that a variety of instructional designs are possible.

What innovations could you use in your situation?

Feedback:
If you agree with Chase (1983) that 'clinical teaching is still one of the most rewarding areas in nursing education' (p. 348) you will find that this activity draws on your creativity and inventiveness.

Matheney (1969) describes two distinct phases, a teacher-led discussion period, followed by a student-centred phase where data for the ensuing clinical assignment were collected and the plans for care reviewed. Mitchell and Krainovich (1982) retained the two-stage pre-conference, emphasizing its value in these terms:

> *Teacher-directed or conference-room phase:*
> The instructor gives additional base line data to each student and discusses overall assignment objectives that relate to the theory covered in class. If, for example, students are on a neurology unit and the topic is genitourinary problems, the instructor has an opportunity to teach from commonalities rather than from a disease model. Drawing on shared problems, students learn to integrate knowledge and apply it to new situations (p. 824).

The authors believe that the importance of the student-centred phase is not understood and that little use is made of it. Rather than proceeding directly to the clinical assignment, Mitchell and Krainovich take the view that additional data-collecting, assessing and planning are necessary and that this should take place in the *student-centred phase*:

> Since students receive baseline data in the pre-conference, they should go directly to the patient to continue data collection and

> assessment before reviewing the chart. This establishes a good work practice and emphasizes the importance of meeting the immediate comfort and safety needs of the patient. Also, students quickly learn that theoretical priorities of patient care established in the conference room may have to be modified when they actually see the patient. For example, a student identified suctioning as the first priority of care for a patient with an artificial airway. When the student saw the patient, he was breathing comfortably, but his Foley catheter had disconnected from the drainage bag. Priorities were adjusted. This system simulates the work situation (p. 824).

Believing that 'innovative approaches to preclinical conferences can maximize the instructor's ability to support and guide the total clinical group', DiRienzo (1983, p. 84) sought a pre-clinical conference strategy which would overcome students' passive, dependent roles in the conference. Small group learning strategies and interaction processes were successful in meeting students' needs for stress reduction but problems remained especially in preparing students for problem-solving in the uncontrollable clinical setting. Eventually a questioning technique was developed to trigger the students' critical thinking. Instead of asking students 'What can you tell us about Mr X'? requiring students to read from their notes, questions became more searching, such as 'Knowing what you do about Mr X, what problems (or decisions, or actions, etc.) do you foresee'? The strategy led to a change in the conduct of the session; the instructor became less active whilst the students became less passive and increasingly independent, not only in the session but throughout the clinical day.

Skurski (1985) has successfully used nursing rounds instead of the traditional pre-conference session in a classroom/conference room setting. The day prior to their clinical practice students are responsible for interviewing their patients, obtaining a health data base, making a nursing diagnosis and planning the nursing actions. With the staff the next morning they listen to the night nurse's report and make changes to their care plans if necessary.

The nursing round commences outside the patient's room with the assigned student giving only the patient's name, age and nursing diagnosis to the group. Further information is given later, the aim being that all students in the group should use their observational skills. After briefly introducing the group and the clinical teacher to the patient, the student explains the diagnosis and nursing care.

Questions, observations and suggestions by the group contribute to the discussion which is held outside the patient's room. Skurski claims that the same amount of time (30 minutes) is spent on this variation of the pre-conference as on the traditional method. The advantages claimed by Skurski are:

> The instructor is able to create a learning atmosphere in which students share with each other as resource persons. In this way decision-making skills can be assessed and desired behaviours reinforced. It is easy to see how this method can show the degree of a student's preparation for clinical practice. . . . Although students are assigned only one client, they have a vicarious experience with several clients. They also learn to assist each other with nursing care and are less hesitant in answering the clients' lights (p. 167).

The problem-based, integrated programme offered in some schools such as Macarthur in Australia has produced a format of clinical experiences fully integrated with the students' problem-solving activities. In Chapter 2 reference was made to situation improvement packages (SIPs) which are actual client problems. Students work with the resource material in the package, and also with clients to arrive at a situation improvement summary. The process represents a cycle of preparation (briefing) clinical practice and reflection/analysis (debriefing).

> As happens in reality, patients' conditions and circumstances change. Therefore students are presented with a series of stimuli known as blocks which constitute a learning 'package' (SIP). The duration of the exploration of one package may vary but always includes one week of related clinical experience (Andersen, 1990b, p. 7).

Clinical assignments take a different form as the students have already carried out problem-based assignments as an on-going activity during the 'blocks' of stimuli. As Andersen (1989) explains:

> The clinical week associated with a SIP provides experiences on themes e.g. oxygen deficiency, related to the focus of the package. It causes students to extend the breadth and depth of concept network development, to consolidate skills and have repeated encounters with their patients. These actual experiences are fed back to the subsequent 'classroom' simulated encounters and stimulate learning issues in their own rights (p. 17).

What can be inferred from the work of the clinical teachers we have cited? From the variety of methods and innovations it is obvious that clinical teachers are striving to be as effective as possible in preparing students for clinical practice. From the modifications of the early model of Matheney, and the later innovations, clinical teachers have adapted briefing sessions to overcome what they perceived as deficiencies in the methods they inherited. In doing so they have shown that traditional classroom teaching is not an appropriate model for preparing students for learning about practice, for a clinical assignment or for a clinical experience.

One further inference can be made, namely, that when 'the action context and the reality of practice determine learning (not the traditional disciplines); . . . when clinical experiences are to be integral to learning, not just illustrative of seemingly more important content; they are valid as initial stimuli of learning' (Andersen, 1990a, p. 6) the result is that a total programme can be designed, integrated and directed toward preparing students for practice.

It is possible that in the present reality of your situation, the constraints of time, staffing, programme design, demands of the institution, climate of the clinical/community facility make innovation impossible. What you require is a departure from the traditional classroom model, but a set of sound guidelines which can be used for either a briefing or a debriefing session.

Reilly and Oermann (1985) provide such a list:

1. At the outset the objectives for the conference should be clarified.

2. The discussion should reflect principles of group process and dynamics.

3. The teacher has an important role in keeping the discussion focused, without dominating it, and providing necessary feedback to learners.

4. The teacher should emphasize periodically the major points made.

5. The atmosphere of the discussion should encourage participation, learner willingness to take risks in responding, and acceptance of different approaches and opinions.

6. Group size should generally be limited to approximately ten to twelve participants to allow for adequate exchange of ideas among them.

7. The physical arrangement should provide for face-to-face discussion.

8. At the conclusion of the conference, a summary should be given by teacher or student of the learning outcomes and applicability to other clinical situations (p. 124).

4.7 PRACTICE-BASED BRIEFING SESSIONS

This section includes the following:

1. self-directed learning;
2. contracting;
3. coaching;
4. questioning;
5. facilitating;
6. preparing for debriefing.

Some of the clinical teacher's frustration in selecting teaching/learning strategies is reflected by Werner-McCullogh and l'Orange when they suggest 'Putting "oomph" into clinical conferences' (1985). Their approaches include problem-solving, nursing rounds, clinical testing and role playing to 'add variety to theoretically based conferences'. Perhaps that is where the problem lies. Is a theoretically based conference synonymous with a briefing session? Can students concentrate on a theory driven briefing when their major motivation is 'I want to know how to cope in clinical'?

Let us consider what teaching/learning strategies can be suggested for a practice-based briefing session.

Activity:
Think of some of the strategies you have used in briefing sessions that you consider worked really well. What did you do and what did the students do? Why do you think those briefing sessions were successful?

Feedback:
Let us start first with what led you to believe that those briefing sessions were successful. Did you ask a colleague to sit in with you to give you feedback? Perhaps you debriefed to a colleague later so that you could go over the session, reflecting on particular parts of the session that were of concern to you or the students. Alternatively you may have recorded the session on audio or video tape

and then asked a colleague to review it with you. Or maybe you used none of these and simply kept a record of your observations during the session. If so, what observations of your students did you make? Were the students alert, quick to ask questions? Did they engage each other in discussion within the group, come up with interesting, different and insightful comments, raise issues for which there was no satisfactory answer and which needed to be addressed by the whole group later, after further information or analysis? Did the students drag their feet when the time came for clinical practice or did they commence with enthusiasm, anticipation and curiosity? Did you feel they were prepared and ready for clinical practice that day?

If those were your observations it can be assumed with safety that you did not choose to give a mini-lecture; that, in fact, your students were active, probably involved in intriguing problems which were relevant to all of them and which were chosen because they would be facing similar problems in the clinical practice to follow.

Self-directed learning

Self-directed learning may also engage the students in issues relevant to their personal growth, clinical skills and understanding of the theoretical base of their practice. Earlier we mentioned the advantages of holding the briefing in a location adjacent to the clinical or community setting. While possibly easier to arrange for clinical than for community placements, the proximity allows students in self-directed learning mode to move back and forth to the clinical setting during the briefing session in order to obtain further information, consult a resource person, read a client's chart or clarify an important or puzzling issue. The freedom offered by self-directed learning assumes a different dimension in clinical teaching. When in doubt in the classroom self-directed learners can fall back on the teacher as the resource and the authority. In the clinical setting, the self-directed learner who has defined learning objectives for practice, and the associated problems to investigate, may find that the teacher is not the authority in that particular problem area. In fact, the resource is the students' existing experience and skills which they are learning to use. If you have tried self-directed learning as a teaching/learning strategy you will agree that the students are highly motivated, learn to take responsibility, learn how to learn and are vigorous in pursuing problems which they themselves have identified as important in learning to nurse.

What role does the clinical teacher have in self-directed learning? Deciding on the amount of freedom to allow students is critical in order to protect clients and to ensure that students have the capability to carry out and complete self-directed clinical practice. Colleagueship, partnership and negotiation are important components of the clinical teacher's role. A degree of trust in the student's ability is necessary, together with a relationship that allows teacher and student frequent reviews of progress to ensure that the objectives are still appropriate, feasible and attainable and the results of the learning and practice are advantageous to all parties.

Contracting

In a similar vein, Sasmor (1984) asked 'Can teaching-learning contracts be used effectively in the practical component of nursing education? The answer is: emphatically, yes!' (p. 171). In addition to the advantages mentioned above, contract learning in clinical experience, (as a form of self-directed learning) fosters the development of desired behaviour and attitudes. According to Sasmor,

> If one assumes that professional nurses are responsible for their own professional development, then one assumes that professional behaviour includes self-analysis/needs assessment, seeking out ways of meeting identified needs and specifying how the achievement of particular goals will be evaluated. That, in essence, is the contracting experience (p. 172).

Coaching

The coaching role which clinical teachers might choose to adopt for tutoring individual students has three distinct, yet overlapping styles: 'follow me!; joint experimentation; hall of mirrors' (Schon, 1988). Adopting a coaching style as a preparation for clinical practice could involve the clinical teacher in a close, rewarding relationship with individual students.

'Follow me!' could be interpreted as 'I will show you how, but then I want you to show me'. This could be something the student has especially requested during the briefing session.

'Joint experimentation' interpreted as 'Let's find out together' in the briefing session could be designing a project to be completed later by students and clinical teacher aimed at finding the meaning of a confusing or complex clinical or practical situation or condition.

'Hall of mirrors' style of coaching, in the briefing session could be interpreted as 'how can we see the client's problem and your intervention from as many perspectives as we can?'

It is unlikely that you would use all of the styles in a single briefing session, and indeed none of the styles may be appropriate for your group of students at their level of experience and learning. The attitude implicit in the two-way coach–student style provides a worthwhile foundation for professional practice where colleagues can give and accept advice, prompting, know-how and feedback. If you have tried to coach rather than to teach in some of your briefing sessions you will have noticed how informal, warm and open the sessions become. Also, the session is unlikely to be focused on 'theoretically based' content, but is highly relevant to the practice to be performed and thus is involving, and prompts students themselves to identify and find the theoretical underpinnings they need to understand that particular practice.

Questioning

Because all of the above modes (problem-based learning, self-directed learning, contracting and coaching) have in common elements of searching, questioning, testing, reviewing, risking, valuing and verifying, a teaching/learning strategy which encourages those cognitive skills is necessary. Certainly techniques of questioning are important in any form of teaching and learning. Craig and Page (1981) observed asking stimulating and challenging questions is one of the most important skills of the clinical teacher. They designed a self-instructional module to assist clinical teachers to use questions calling on more than a simple recall of knowledge and instead generating questions at each level of Bloom's Taxonomy. They claim some success but report that only one fifth of teachers who used the module actually asked higher level questions.

Certainly there is merit in preparing a number of questions designed to stimulate students to think more deeply than simple recall of factual content. There are important differences in the type of questions used in the classroom and those used by the clinical teacher. Stimulating students to uncover the hidden meaning of their clinical experiences is to point them to the 'hidden curriculum' of clinical learning. Some students will miss it altogether, being concerned only with the task to be completed. The expertise of the clinical teacher in awakening students to the otherwise unrecognized insights and discoveries to be made lies in skills of questioning and facilitation.

Facilitating

Many clinical teachers who have included problem-based and self-directed learning in their programme claim that their questioning skills need to be further developed. Moreover, the skill of shifting the students' dependence from the teacher to themselves is more difficult than it seems.

> . . . the most significant variable in the effective implementation of problem-based learning is the skill of the tutor as a facilitator. In problem-based tutorials, the student's skills of critical thinking are developed by constantly challenging their assumptions; their understanding, by constantly challenging their knowledge base; their self-directed learning skills, by constantly challenging their ability to identify their learning needs and ability to assess accurately their own performances. It is by providing these challenges that the tutor facilitates the student's learning (Little, 1987, cited in McMillan and Dwyer (1989).

McMillan and Dwyer (1989), citing Little (1987), shed further light on the facilitator of learning in problem-based clinical teaching. A different kind of questioning is needed, structured and sequenced so that students are led through their own paths of thinking to show how they came to a certain conclusion. In turn, other students are involved in the process, challenging critically the statements each makes. It goes without saying that in order to facilitate effectively in this manner, clinical teachers need to review their own reasoning processes.

How stressful is the facilitation process for individual students? Obviously, for the method to be successful, a supporting, nurturing, understanding as well as challenging environment is necessary.

An example of an episode of facilitation in a briefing session is given below, extracted from the tape 'Critical Incidents in Clinical Teaching' (1988).

The facilitation skills of the clinical teacher are exemplified in series of challenging questions. In sequence the skills are:

1. assisting clarification;
2. facilitating exploration;
3. exploring approaches;
4. encouraging analysis;
5. promoting interpretation;
6. checking meaning;

7. clarifying perceptions;
8. prompting understanding.

The scene: The students are half way through a period of four weeks clinical practice which accompanies a module on orthopaedic nursing. The clinical teacher and students have together selected the clinical assignments for the clinical practice session. Just before commencing the assignment for the day the student approaches the clinical teacher with the request that she be moved to another clinical placement. They meet in the briefing room.

The student explains that she is having difficulties and repeats her request for another placement.

Clarification

C.T.: Yes, that could be arranged but it seems we need to clarify what it actually is about orthopaedics or orthopaedic patients that is the problem. What about orthopaedics as a specialty, is that a difficulty?

St.: Oh no – I understand orthopaedic nursing and have done stacks of assessments of orthopaedic conditions and I feel confident – I feel I know it quite well.

Exploration

C.T.: Alright, so is it working with orthopaedic patients that's the problem?

St.: No. It's not orthopaedic patients. I get on well with most of them and I have no problems in caring for them – it's . . . just . . . one of them, . . . Clive.

C.T.: I see, let's look at Clive as an orthopaedic patient, is that the problem?

St.: Well, his osteo is chronic so he's got a low grade fever and a bit of pain sometimes – he's bored and restless – and although he's young and generally healthy he's beginning to develop some of the complications of immobility.

C.T.: Is their anyone else in ward in his age group?

St.: Yes, but they don't behave like him!

C.T.: So is it Clive's behaviour as an orthopaedic patient that's the problem.

St.: No, I guess not.

C.T.: Well, what is it then?

St.: [*Hesititating*] He's just a really difficult person and it's very hard trying to nurse him.

Encouraging analysis

C.T.: I see – well that's not an uncommon problem in nursing. It happens to most of us from time to time that we encounter patients that are 'difficult' and it's very awkward for us to care for them. But I really want to get back to analysing what it is that's happening here. Do you have any thoughts about this?

St.: No – not really, it's not the same way as assessing the medical or nursing condition, is it?

C.T.: No it's not, but it's just as important a process as the assessment process.

St.: I can vaguely remember something from social and behavioural science that touched on this kind of problem, but I guess I could go and look it up.

Promoting interpretation

C.T.: You could – and you could do that later. Let's start with the problem. I want to try and work out what it is about Clive that makes it so difficult for you here. You can tie it into the theory later.

St.: Well, we're very very different! Worlds apart. How do you analyse that?

C.T.: You could start by looking at Clive as a person and at you as a person. How do you see Clive?

St.: Well, he's a bikie, looks like one and acts like one – he's rude, rough, loud, has tattoos all over . . . he's 20 and still reads comics . . . and his language!

Checking meaning

C.T.: Those impressions add up to a set of symbols that tend to stereotype Clive – do they have symbolic significance for you?

St.: Yes, I guess they do – I do react to them.

C.T.: Alright, let's leave that for a moment. How do you think Clive sees you?

St.: Oh, that I speak with an upper class accent, that I'm stuck up – that I'm better than him – all of that and a lot more that's unrepeatable.

C.T.: Alright. [*Draws a large circle on paper.*] Just imagine that this is Clive . . . you seem to be reacting to a whole set of cues that place Clive in a certain group in a particular environment. Right?

St.: Yes.

Clarifying perceptions

C.T.: This is you over here [*draws another circle*] and Clive is probably doing exactly the same thing. Responding to you as representing a group in society that generally looks down on people like Clive and probably fears them too. [*Draws arrows to Clive and the opposite way to Sharon.*] How do you suppose that influences the way you react to each other?

St.: I guess we're just reacting to all those external cues and not seeing each other as people with individual characteristics and needs.

Prompting understanding

C.T.: Do you remember learning about that in class?

St.: Yes, I think so.

C.T.: What's the theory called?

St.: Umm . . . Symbolic interaction . . . I think.

C.T.: That's right. Do you remember what it's about?

St.: Yes, it tries to explain what the influences are between people who are trying to communicate. Although I've never had to apply it before.

The briefing moves into prompting the student to plan the changes she would now make, following the insight she has gained into the problem.

Preparing for debriefing the experience

Briefing and debriefing sessions are part of a continuous process. Debriefing 'cold' after clinical experience without the advantages of looking ahead to the possible areas for analysis is less than profitable for students learning. While free association of ideas and reactions in the group can be cathartic, the purpose of the debriefing session is to derive as much from the clinical experience as is possible.

The focus for debriefing after clinical practice needs to be established in the briefing. Students must be alerted to the need to reflect upon their activities and to be ready to analyse some of the critical areas of their practice.

They can then be encouraged to contract with the clinical teacher for components of their practice to be observed and analysed during the debriefing session. The system devised for supervision of teacher-education students (Turney *et al.*, 1982) includes a series of teaching skills for the pre-observation period. These are directed toward the student-teacher explaining the nature of the lesson to be given and the aspects upon which comment is sought and analysis requested. Some of these teaching skills are similar in purpose to those for preparation of nursing students for the clinical assignment (p. 79) above. However, because of the uncontrollable and unpredictable environment of the clinical nursing situation, not all the possibilities available in practice can be anticipated. Additional teaching skills are needed. Preparing students to learn from experience in such a rich environment means helping them to realize that what they expect in clinical may be different from what they will find. According to Benner and Wrubel (1982a), examining the difference between expectations and reality is critical in clinical learning. When this is not done, clinical situations do not qualify as experience. The benefits of so examining clinical experience is in the development of clinical knowledge.

4.8 THE ROLE OF THE CLINICAL TEACHER IN THE BRIEFING SESSION

Activity:
Although some of the roles will be similar to those of the lab, the different purposes of briefing and the smaller group of students will influence the way you enact your role. If you want the briefing session to reflect the major issues raised in this chapter, what will be your roles?

Feedback:
If your students are to learn how to learn in clinical your role as empathic *supporter* will include;

1. helping them to identify their concerns;
2. providing ways to reduce stress;
3. encouraging them to identify their learning needs;
4. developing independent problem-solving skills.

If your students' clinical assignments are to be effective your role as *planner* will include:

1. visiting clients to seek their involvement;
2. negotiating with clinical staff;
3. fitting clinical resources to individual students;
4. anticipating problems;
5. allowing for contingencies;

6. assessing individual students' readiness;
7. recognizing strengths and advising on improvement.

If your students are to gain from the experience your role as their *coach* will include:

1. demonstrating a working relationship of openness and trust so that you and the students are partners;
2. learning from and with each other; preparing for collaboration and co-operation.

If you are to encourage independence through self-directed learning in clinical your role as *resource person* will include:

1. uncovering your students' intentions and expectations;
2. encouraging students' initiatives;
3. rewarding independent performance;
4. supporting effort;
5. stimulating creativity.

If you are to support contracting as a strategy to develop your students' sense of responsibility your *professional role-model* will include demonstrating your own self-analysis and responses to the challenges of being a professional.

If your students are to develop practice-based knowledge your role as *facilitator* will include:

1. preparing students to examine critically their assumptions, knowledge base and attitudes in the clinical setting;
2. preparing challenges for students to understand what they will see, do and experience in clinical.

If your students are to prepare for the debriefing session to follow clinical practice your role as an *inquirer* will include:

1. alerting students to recognize in their everyday clinical experiences questions for critical analysis;
2. encouraging students to note whether their expectations differ from what actually happens;
3. planning for co-investigation of questions identified by students;
4. offering availability to discuss meanings as well as concrete practice;
5. demonstrating an inquiry approach to own role.

5

Learning through clinical practice

There is an assumption in the clinical learning cycle (Figure 5.1) that the clinical teacher and students proceed together from the briefing session into the clinical or community setting. In many programmes that is certainly the case. In other programmes the reality is very different. Several constraints operate: programme constraints, where the curriculum structure separates the theoretical component from the clinical component so that few classroom teachers are also clinical teachers; economic constraints and limited funding for the clinical teaching programme; logistic constraints due to increasing numbers of students and pressure on student to teacher ratios. These have all contributed to the re-consideration of the process of clinical teaching. Some programmes have sought solutions in the addition of clinical teachers whose responsibilities are for teaching only in the clinical/community setting itself. Other programmes have implemented mentor or preceptorship systems, involving clinical staff in student teaching.

The focus of this chapter is the skills employed by the clinical teacher who is in direct contact with students in the clinical/community setting. It will be assumed that students have had a range of experiences in preparation for the clinical teaching task and that all have had a briefing session. Some teachers may have advantages in knowing the clients, others in knowing the students; some in knowing both. It will be assumed that all clinical teachers are familiar with the programme of the school, the clinical teaching module the students are currently studying and the nature of the briefing sessions they have attended.

By the end of the chapter you will have identified a range of clinical teaching/learning styles and skills, assessed the clinical en-

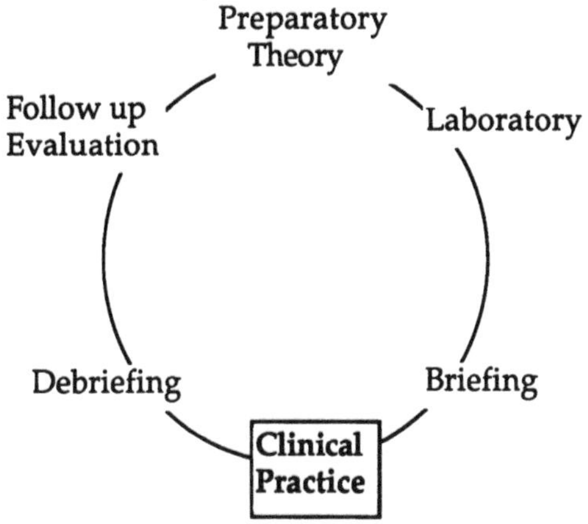

Figure 5.1 Clinical learning cycle: clinical practice.

vironment for its influence on learning, reviewed the types of clinical assignments in relation to the purposes of clinical teaching in your programme and explored the value of the students' clinical experience.

Activity:
No one would doubt the importance of the clinical/community setting for students' learning. There is less agreement on what it is that clinical teachers are doing when students are in the practice setting. Clinical teachers themselves are often unsure what is expected of them. Take a few moments to think of a 'typical' clinical practice day with a group of six to eight students. What are your usual activities? Make a list of everything you do, and try to include the everyday activities even though they might seem unimportant to you. Then try scanning the list to find groups of activities that fit together. What inferences can you make about your function as a clinical teacher?

Feedback:
You may have placed at the top of the list the practical day-to-day, and hour-to-hour demands of clinical teaching, such as:

1. making sure each student is ready to proceed;
2. keeping an eye on students who could be in difficulty;
3. noting the changes in patients and in the ward or agency 'climate';

4. anticipating possible concerns of students *vis-à-vis* distressed, disturbed or complex conditions of clients;
5. reviewing assignments and plans with students as situations change during the day;
6. balancing the time spent with each student in relation to the location of students in different wards or departments;
7. keeping alert to happenings in the area that could constitute a valuable learning opportunity and gathering students to witness or to participate;
8. being ready to guide students when they are unsure;
9. conferring and negotiating with clinical/community staff and facilitating interpersonal relationships;
10. weighing up the progress of students in the last hour of practice to make sure each student will be able to finish on time.

Your list may also deal with what you do in those extended periods you have with individual students, such as

- supporting
- observing
- guiding
- facilitating
- caring
- inquiring
- researching
- evaluating
- resourcing
- instructing

These can be broadly categorized as 'active teaching'.

What possible inferences could you draw about your function as a clinical teacher? Taking the first set of activities (1–10) we could say they represent

1. management activities to ensure smooth implementation of the clinical programme throughout the day, which together resemble an unwritten 'maintenance routine';
2. contingency management which anticipates difficulties, impediments in progress, and considers the implications of changes in the environment which could affect students' practice.

The active teaching category suggests several domains:

1. teaching/learning activities, implemented according to cues from students; supporting, observing, guiding, facilitating, resourcing;

2. triad activities where student, patient and teacher are involved in caring and instructing according to cues from patients;
3. personal/professional activities such as discussions with clinical staff to keep up to date, orienting to new equipment, inquiring into puzzling or conflicting situations, researching clinical issues and problems;
4. programme-related activities such as evaluations of students' performance, devising and implementing clinical assessment schedules, advising on curriculum implementation issues, such as the effectiveness of the relation of theoretical to clinical components.

What value to you is the identification and analysis of your function as a clinical teacher? There are many aspects of your work that remain unrecognized and therefore much of what you do is undervalued. When the traditions of classroom teaching tend to permeate clinical teaching it is little wonder that clinical teaching is considered to be a simple off-shoot of the skills of instruction, with an occasional demonstration, and a majority of 'elbow supervision'.

A helpful exercise you could try is to keep a log of the time you spend each day in each area of the categories of clinical teaching you have identified. You could find that you want to add extra dimensions as you uncover other activities you have previously taken for granted.

Students often wonder what you will actually be doing while you are with them. Their previous experiences in other clinical areas and with other clinical teachers leads them to wonder whether you will observe them continuously, supervise, correct, evaluate, or take part in the care. Their assumptions about your function might not accord with what you intend and could easily lead to misunderstandings and unrealizable expectations. If you have been in the briefing session with these students you would have had opportunities for explaining what you intend to do. It is a sound idea to be explicit about your function, as it relates to them on each day, for example: 'You know that today I'll be your back-up if you're not sure, not to take over, but to stand-by if you need it. I won't be evaluating you today but I will be observing those special things you asked me to look for, in the briefing session'.

You could also anticipate students' concerns by telling them how you plan to spend the time with each of them individually, where you will be and how they can contact you when necessary. You might also wish to be explicit about your plans by letting students know your objectives for the day, and what you plan to achieve through the activities you and the students will be involved in. As well as offering reassurance, your involvement with them as a colleague is a powerful motivator for professional performance.

Activity:
While it is true that there has been a lack of clarity about what clinical teachers do, there is even more uncertainty about how they do it. Why not inquire into your own teaching to describe how you work with your students? Try taking the list of activities under teaching/learning, above, and when next you are engaged in any one of them, make mental notes of what happened, then as soon as you can, describe what took place. You could talk into a tape recorder while still in the vicinity, or choose some other way of recording. You could then use the information for identifying your clinical teaching style and for comparing the major ways you teach with some of your colleagues.

Feedback:
Some research studies have described students' opinions about effective and ineffective clinical teaching behaviour but the scarcity of research into the activities of clinical teaching and the lack of opportunities for 'sitting in' to observe clinical teaching have resulted in a web of mystique surrounding the clinical teaching encounter. You could begin to dispel the mystique, in the interests of recognition of the full sweep of clinical teaching, by persuading your colleagues to explore how they support, facilitate, observe (or any other active teaching activity) and then together present the information as a discussion paper to your school and/or institution, and later, to a wider readership through a journal.

Let us pursue some clinical teaching styles in each of the activities we listed as active teaching above.

5.1 SUPPORTING

Activity:
Your style of supporting students has probably evolved out of many occasions where you have responded to 'pick up' a nervous student or to jolly along another who is keen but timid. Compare your experiences with those below.

Feedback:
Support as a teaching/learning skill has undergone many changes since the days when students were expected to be seen and not

heard and when any indication of needing support was a sign of unsuitability for a career in nursing. Consequently, teachers in the clinical setting were considered 'weak' if they 'gave in' to students who allowed their anxiety to show. Students and teachers now regard giving support as an essential component of nursing, and as students experience many different ways support can be given to them, they, in turn, learn how to recognize the need for support in their patients and peers.

We will look at support in the following ways:

1. need for support;
2. support in specific episodes of learning;
3. support as a teaching/learning process;
4. types of social support.

Need for support

The importance of assuring students of your support cannot be overestimated. Windsor (1987) reports that although they might have performed without problems in the lab, when students were performing a procedure with a patient for the first time they wanted the teacher to be present because they were not sure what they were doing.

You might consider that your students have been supported sufficiently already and can go straight ahead. If they have been present during the report and hand-over you might have had opportunity for some support at that time. Remembering that their concentration will be on their clinical assignments, the support, if in the form of directions, needs to be brief. Remembering also that students new to an area need more support than usual, you might also consider that a personal assurance that you will be in close contact is necessary. Kleehammer *et al.* (1990) report on students' perceptions of anxiety-producing situations in the clinical setting. Four major themes emerged; 'negative interaction with the instructor was mentioned most often, with student anxiety concerning nursing procedures, fear of making mistakes, and the initial clinical experience as second, third and fourth' (p. 186).

Support in specific episodes of learning

In one of the rare studies of the clinical teacher in action, Carr (1983) reports observations of the ways clinical teachers support students in specific episodes of learning. Compare how you support students with the following:

> acting with and reacting to a student by giving time to the student to work with the familiar and known first, making sure to be there during the less familiar [Carr gives an example of the teacher's estimation that the student will be unsure in caring for a dying patient]
>
> thinking through an activity first alone, then with the student
>
> identifying and strengthening initiatives of behaviour which students might not realize is commendable
>
> assuring and reassuring struggling students that there can be an attainable solution
>
> showing faith and trust in students' capabilities
>
> rewarding a student by accepting and adopting a student's decision (Carr, 1983, p. 294).

Support as a teaching/learning process

Contractual support may be arranged between the student and clinical teacher and/or a clinical specialist. A three-way contract allows inclusion of the expert clinical or community practitioner in a special area to have definite responsibility in the student's learning. The contract may be verbal or written and usually made prior to practice, in a briefing session, or immediately before a clinical assignment by all parties. The contract includes, for example, agreements about the roles the participants accept in relation to the student's assignment; agreements about the limits of performance; agreements about the feedback each requires of the other. Contractual support enables arrangements to be made which free the student from anxiety about being left without necessary direction, information or support in a distressful or difficult situation, yet allows some opportunities for individual decision-making and creativity.

Informed support is preferable to bland general comments which convey platitudes and a lack of interest in and perception of, the students' individual effort and developing practice style. Detailed knowledge and expertise of the clinical specialty is required so that specific comments are given to accompany the progress of an interaction or an intervention, or the initiation of a painful or distressing procedure. When support is linked specifically to the student's practice, for example, giving feedback to affirm accuracy of specific actions, remarking on the appropriateness of specific initiatives or praising a demonstration of exceptional caring, the student's experience of success in practice is reinforced. When support is linked specifically to the student's learning, for example, recognizing instances of understanding that show the student's grasp of principles underlying an action, a behaviour or a patient's condition; recognizing the student's progress in learning by expecting an insightful answer to a penetrating question; or praising the struggling steps taken to learn how single episodes of practice relate to a wider context, the student's perception of progress in learning is sharpened.

Non-verbal support by gestures can be particularly powerful in reinforcing desirable activities. When it is more appropriate to avoid verbal expressions, the clinical teacher can support the student's intentions or actions by nodding, facial expression, eye to eye contact, gestures and stance. It is important to remember how one's own insecurity as a student was influenced for the better or otherwise, by the body language of a teacher or qualified practitioner. Although non-verbal, the cues picked up by nervous students are unmistakable. On the other hand, some over-anxious students may misinterpret non-verbal cues and require more substantial indications of support.

Silent support or 'the supporting presence' offers neither approval nor disapproval but simply shows the student that the commitment to 'stand by' has been honoured until the student indicates that the clinical teacher's presence is no longer required. Flagler *et al.* (1988) in 'Clinical teaching is more than evaluation alone' call this support, 'benevolent presence' by simply 'being there' for the student and 'not holding the student responsible for seeking help' (p. 347). Students often believe that seeking help is an indication of incompetence as a learner and are reluctant to signal when and for what they need the clinical teacher's presence.

When you know the students well enough you can support them according to the needs for support they expressed during the briefing session and as you or individual students identify additional needs during the course of the practice period. Students also support one another to a quite considerable degree. Often they are in the best position to know the real source of anxiety and can give realistic support from a peer perspective. Encouraging peer support is worthwhile in all stages of the clinical learning cycle and paves the way for professional-colleague openness in relationships as graduates.

Types of social support

One way of summarizing the issues for the clinical teacher is to cite the four categories of social support identified by House (1981):

1. *Emotional support* by showing concern and listening; providing affection and love; and being trustworthy. Enhancing students' self-esteem and sense of well-being is influential in helping them come to terms with the realities and stresses of learning in clinical practice.
2. *Appraisal support* by giving affirmation and feedback. The urgency of 'knowing how I'm going' expressed so often by students indicates the need for and benefit of specific, immediate and concrete informed feedback.
3. *Informational support* through advice, information and assistance with the steps in working through a clinical problem or the uncertainty and ambiguity of a community assignment.
4. *Instrumental support* through the availability of resources such as appropriate clinical or community assignments and access to personnel in addition to the clinical teacher (adapted from House, 1981, quoted in Smythe, 1984).

5.2 OBSERVING

Whether the setting for clinical practice is a clinic, a ward, a patient's home, a community health centre, or other agency, it is usually a rich context for observing human behaviour and organizational climate. The environmental climate for teaching and learning is the topic of a later section in this chapter. While aware of the importance of assessing the impact of the environment on learning and teaching, the clinical teacher is concerned mainly with observation of the learning triad, student, patient (client, family, group, or other face-to-face focus) and self.

Activity:
No doubt your approach to observing your students will have developed over time and, of course, will change according to the needs of the students and the characteristics of their clinical assignments. What ways of observing students' performance have you found best meet your needs for information and your students' needs for assistance?

Feedback:
Some students may have indicated to you the specific areas of performance they want you to observe so that their analysis in the debriefing session has a definite focus. Other students may be ambivalent, wanting you to be there at critical points just in case there is a difficulty, but not wanting you to stay when they are more assured. Obviously, both you and the students have different purposes in observing clinical performance. Discussion prior to the clinical assignment is therefore preferable to avoid unplanned periods of observation where there can be misunderstandings about the reason for extended periods with particular students.

(Turney *et al.*, 1982) point to the value of 'focus points' in determining what can feasibly be observed during one episode of practice. Smyth (1984) also offers helpful comments on the observation of teacher-education students which are useful for the clinical teacher in nursing education. It is important, Smyth says, that the objective of the session is to describe performance rather than to evaluate it. In that way, judgement on the performance is suspended until the student has a chance later to interpret the clinical teacher's description from her/his own perspective.

Focus on the student

When your students have signalled that they want you to observe a specific performance (for example, as they are interacting with a newly admitted patient, performing a dressing likely to be painful, or supporting a family of a terminally ill person); they know that when you appear there is a definite purpose in an extended period of observation. The unspecified hovering that students find so threatening is avoided. On the other hand, there are advantages for the student in the clinical teacher being a sensitive, unsolicited observer, able, to the student's surprise, to give feedback on a particularly commendable performance, or to point to where desired improvement could occur.

Another occasion when focused observation is advantageous, and in fact, essential, is where the student and clinical teacher have agreed that the teacher will intervene, if necessary, during a difficult, complex or hazardous activity in the care of a client. When the method of intervention has been agreed upon prior to the event (e.g., by a form of words, gestures or actions) the patient is not alarmed, and the student is protected from the clinical teacher 'taking over' and assuming control.

Focus on the patient

Students develop skills in noting the changes occurring in the patient's physical condition and illness stages. Their skills in matching physiological signs with accompanying behaviour changes is an indication of their advancement in clinical knowledge. Similarly, students become skilled in noting obvious signs of fear, distress, withdrawal and other overt indications of the emotional responses of patients. However, more subtle cues of response and reactions within an episode of clinical practice are often missed. Beginning students, particularly, often find difficulty in managing the competing demands of the situation for their attention. Concern to perform accurately and competently and to follow guidelines and rules to the letter tend to take priority. Senior students also need to be alerted to the often overlooked signals from patients (or clients and families in community situations) such as:

1. confusion about an explanation and too embarrassed to ask for clarity;
2. exhaustion after a supposedly non-taxing treatment;
3. misunderstanding of an explanation given in technical language by an enthusiastic student;
4. facial expression or gesture indicating 'unasked questions';
5. readiness (or alternatively, absence of readiness) to learn about the illness or treatment;
6. missed cues signalling impending change;
7. cues indicating changes in the stages of the student/teacher relationship, for example, threat, trust, defensiveness.

Focusing on own performance

In many respects clinical teaching is a private activity, screened from public view. In classroom teaching observation of teaching is possible (and often welcomed), but in clinical teaching the inclusion of the observer can be intrusive. In the clinical setting for reasons of the patient's privacy, the student's and teacher's vulnerability and the purely practical reasons of space and comfort, an extra person in the teaching environment is not usually desirable.

Clinical teachers who want to find out about their performance can ask students for their opinions and also the patient, whose perspective often provides valuable insights. Reports of surveys of student opinion (such as O'Shea and Parsons, 1979; Windsor, 1987;

Flagler *et al.*, 1988) show how students consider the clinical teacher helps and hinders their learning.

How can you observe your own performance? In a recent workshop clinical teachers were asked what they wanted to know about their clinical teaching performance. Some of their responses are listed below. We have left them verbatim, but have grouped them under self, students and programme. Why not take time to think about what it is that you want to know about your performance? Make a list then compare it with the following. What I want to know about my performance is:

1. Am I challenging enough?
2. Do students perceive me as a facilitator of learning?
3. Am I a suitable instrument for the students to learn from?
4. How effective am I in all the 'layers' of clinical?
5. Have I helped them understand nursing from the client's perspective?
6. How successful are my interpersonal skills, between students, staff and patients?
7. Does my clinical teaching fit with students' overall picture of nursing and experience?
8. Have I given the students enough support from their perspective and from mine?
9. Am I preparing students for the workplace?
10. Am I following learning models?
11. Is it meeting students needs, curriculum needs and objectives of the session?

The participants then explored how they could obtain this information, that is, how they could answer their own questions. A network of colleagues was formed, comprising those willing to observe another's clinical teaching if possible and feasible. Members of the network also agreed to debrief each other after a clinical teaching session, either face to face, or by listening to an audio-taped recording of the session. Others took up a suggestion of making a quick pocket-note of observations of their actions as soon as possible, (such as, missed an opportunity for . . . ; explanation – good – but check principle; fumbled that direction . . . and so on). Others saw value in noting their feelings in association with a specific action. Momentary reactions are often forgotten soon after; if feelings, say, of tension, excitement, anger, compassion, humour can be recalled and related to what was happening at the time, valuable insights can be gained into how to change unsuccessful strategies, or to adopt satisfactory steps into one's repertoire of skills.

Interestingly, one of the workshop participants asked: 'What indicators can I use to give me a realistic idea of my skills?' Carpenito and Duespohl advise a method of self-evaluation that clinical teachers could use to review their instructional practices. Using Rogerian concepts of empathy, congruence and positive regard, questions relating to each concept have been devised for self-evaluation (Carpenito and Duespohl, 1985, p. 21). The questions relating to empathy are:

1. Are my expectations realistic regarding student preparation the night before clinical practice?
2. Am I sensitive to students' other problems (ill child, need to work)?
3. Would I like myself as a clinical teacher?

Those relating to congruence are:

1. Do I share some of myself with my students?
2. Do students see me as exclusively interested only in nursing?
3. Do I share my mistakes and limitations with students?
4. Do students see me as real and human or stiff and contrived?

The questions relating to positive regard are:

1. Am I afraid to allow students to practice without direct supervision?
2. How do I respond when students challenge me?
3. How do I respond when students make an error?
4. Do I criticize students in the presence of others?
5. Do I treat students in the same manner as I do my professional colleagues?

5.3 GUIDING

While there may be occasions when it will be necessary to demonstrate or instruct in the clinical setting it is more usual for students to have been well prepared beforehand and the need is more for guidance than reteaching what has already been learned.

Activity:
In your explorations of your teaching those actions that suggest you are leading, directing, influencing, motivating, advising and coun-

selling suggest that you are guiding. Your actual style could take the form of non-directive leading, or on the other hand of giving specific advice and direction towards a particular outcome. Try comparing your style with the following examples.

Guiding self-directed students

You have probably found that the guidance of students in the clinical setting actually begins much earlier. In fact, if in the early stages of the clinical learning cycle learners have been encouraged to be self-directed during lab exercises and briefing they will usually seek guidance when they perceive it to be necessary. For example 'I'm not sure how to proceed with Mr X today because his medications have changed and I'm not sure of the indications of reactions to these particular drugs, nor how to interpret his present signs and symptoms'. Guidance from the clinical teacher might take the form of prompting the student to identify where the information can be obtained and from whom; the steps she/he would take to determine the seriousness of the client's condition, the reasoning underlying the interpretations made, and finally, the action if any to be taken. Students say they need the clinical teacher to think of things that might never occur to them (Windsor, 1987), but in guiding students, the teacher prompts by relevant questions, rather than giving the answers. Remember that preparation for self-directed learning in the briefing session (p. 109) emphasized that students are learning to use their own resources of experience and skills.

Guiding students in learning while they are 'doing'

You may have had difficulty in guiding students in learning while they are 'doing'. 'What I do, I know' is a familiar phrase and its basic truth is not disputed, but if it simply means knowing how to do a certain thing through and through, what is it that is being learned? Is it learning a process or an activity; or is it a way of approach to making clients comfortable, or solving problems, or linking past knowledge with present observations? Are students able to say what they are learning while they are doing? How can the clinical teacher guide students during the 'doing' components of the assignment?

Greaves (1979) believes that 'individual procedures' can be 'learning events' if the clinical teacher guides the student in keeping technicalities flexible, adopting creative solutions to individual patients and above all, practising within a total care concept. Guiding students in how to see the numerous aspects involved in one caring episode contributes to a successful performance and also to the student's progress in professional development. There would be little disagreement among clinical teachers that there is a thinking component as well as a doing component in such activities as giving medications and injections, making an assessment, doing a difficult dressing or reading monitors. At the same time Greaves is emphasizing that the guidance of students involves not only the 'content' of the particular activity but its extension into the framework of the patient's situation and surroundings. In other words, unless the actions are learned in the context of the whole situation for the patient and the student, 'learning by doing' can be limited to learning the steps in a series of isolated skills. Put another way, there is rarely so simple a thing as 'learning by doing' as, until the action is habitual and requires no further thinking through all the steps involved (for example swimming, riding a bicycle, typewriting), the 'doer' is also thinking, feeling and experiencing.

Guiding students in a competency-based programme

If you are guiding students in a programme based on competencies which have been identified by the faculty as a whole you may find that, as well as the advantages of clarity in the skills and standards the students are to attain, there are disadvantages if the competencies are not submitted to regular review and revision. Darbyshire *et al.* (1990) found that there was support for the view that competency-based approaches should be viewed critically, and suggested competencies which reflect caring skills and the healing relationship. The concepts are not new in nursing practice but have been expressed as competencies infrequently because of the difficulty in identifying the associated skills which can be part of assessable and measurable performance.

Derbyshire acknowledges the problems but believes students can be guided through a set of competencies which encourage students to view caring holistically. For example, the profile of a competency in the healing relationship is phrased as 'the healing relationship creates a climate for, and establishes a commitment to, healing' (p. 74).

The four levels of performance correspond to four years of an undergraduate programme:

Level 1: identifies the factors necessary to maintain the wholeness and uniqueness of each individual and the components of caring which can support this,

Level 2: is attentive to the needs of individual patients and is developing a range and understanding of own caring practices,

Level 3: fosters hope for patients by helping them interpret and understand their illness and emotions and helps them to use social, emotional or spiritual support,

Level 4: enhances patients' dignity, worth and uniqueness through the demonstration of a consistently involved caring stance and combines intuitive caring skills with a knowledge of relevant research.

(Darbyshire *et al.*, 1990, p. 74)

Guiding students in this competency-based programme includes assisting students to recognize their personal abilities in a healing relationship, modelling when and how a healing relationship can best be developed, encouraging reflective diaries, recording situations significant for them and frequent self-assessments. In addition, guidance in the form of relating to the students in a 'consistently involved caring stance' is important in showing a genuine, personal acceptance of the concepts in this approach.

Guiding students in a concept-based programme

If you are teaching in a concept-based programme the pattern of clinical teaching and learning includes guiding the students in extending and expanding their basic concepts to include the observations, interpretations and insights they discover as they practice. Prompting, questioning and challenging become accepted methods of guidance.

For example, the concept of mobility can be extended to include observations made and experiences of an individual patient in clinical which show the implications of immobility: status, social isolation, physical limitations, physiological complications, structural deformities, and so on. The concept can be further extended to include responses in the form of nursing actions: increasing movements, through passive and active exercises, encouraging involvement in social activities, monitoring physical and structural signs and symptoms, and lastly, suggesting innovative care for these conditions. Having extended the concept the student can then be guided to analyse the wider concept to determine how it could apply to new and different situations.

Guiding students in a problem-based programme

Similarly, if you are teaching in a problem-based programme, based on observation and inquiry, review and researching, again through prompting, questioning and challenging, while students are 'doing', is an expected form of guidance and a learning strategy for students which will become habit forming and eventually part of their everyday professional practice. Taking students through the steps in their observations, assumptions, conclusions and decisions based on their actual experiences, brings to life the simulated problems they have worked with in the lab or the briefing session. Students need guidance in the form of 'leading' them through questions about their problem-solving. As a way of linking theory to practice, the process is demanding for students and teacher alike. It is a process which in its questioning is intellectual, while its subject is a practical 'doing' act. Guiding students through this process requires particular skill to encourage students through a series of sequential, interesting questions so that they will learn to integrate their practical and theoretical knowledge into the outcome, which is clinical knowledge. Sensitivity is needed to distinguish when students respond best to an earnest inquisitorial manner or to a more quizzical 'jollying along' approach.

Guiding students by giving feedback

Giving feedback while students are performing in clinical practice presents invaluable opportunities for guiding individual students. You and the student may decide that you will be present for a particular performance, to give feedback on specific aspects identified beforehand (as well as others that you may notice and need to be corrected at the time). One of the first steps is to provide explanation to the patient first, seeking permission and co-operation and possible involvement in the feedback session. There are likely to be pauses when you will comment on the specific action you are observing, or ask the student to explain how or why he/she is going to proceed in a certain way. Sharing information about the performance in this way is different from giving advice as it leaves the student free to decide what to do. Checking the decision with both you and the patient provides feedback to the student on his/her judgement and allows rethinking if necessary.

Timing the feedback to avoid errors but to allow the student enough opportunity to use individual skill and intuition requires sensitive observation and a degree of trust and genuine concern for the student's development and the patient's welfare and safety. Guiding the student by giving feedback is, in fact, 'giving away skills' – your skills – to the student. In essence, you are guiding by leading 'behind' the student, placing your hand on his/hers at times to transfer the amount of pressure to be used in massage, or 'listening' with the student to body sounds through monitors, or 'seeing' with the student fine discriminations of change in colour or expression.

5.4 FACILITATING

There are numbers of styles of 'facilitating' which seem to be tied to particular programs and philosophies of learning. Of course, personal beliefs about teaching and learning are at the centre of styles of facilitation.

Activity:
You may have developed a style yourself which you have found satisfying. It is interesting to consider the influence of one's personal style on our own and our students' behaviour. There are several examples below. After examining each one, add your own personal style with examples from your own teaching.

Feedback:
While all of the styles of facilitation overlap and interact in clinical teaching, for the purposes of identifying the issues more sharply we will look at two major styles of particular relevance to clinical teachers:

1. Inter-personal
2. Responsive

Inter-personal style

Rogers (1983) in *Freedom to Learn for the 80's*, suggests that facilitators need to be able to respond to the feelings of the learner, as they explore a learning experience. He claims it is also important that the facilitator recognizes his/her own feelings. As the student moves from exploration into understanding, the facilitator responds to the content the student is struggling with. Finally, when the learner's focus is action, the facilitator moves into guiding further development of the student's knowledge and actions.

The following lists some of the ways clinical teachers use an interpersonal style of facilitation:

1. showing interest in the student as a person;
2. taking a personal interest in recognizing individual effort and progress;
3. being understanding and non-judgemental about students' unwarranted anxieties;
4. making students feel free to ask questions and to seek help without fear of loss of confidence, esteem or grades;
5. showing confidence in individual students, giving positive reinforcement;
6. promoting action and discussion about patient care, manipulating the experience to allow students to experience success;
7. reinforcing the expectation of success;
8. fostering students' positive self-confidence.

It is interesting to note that Carr (1983) found in her study an intensely personal style of clinical teaching.

> The teacher's preferred mode of operation was so much a part of the individual teacher that, over time, methods of teaching became increasingly inseparable and indistinguishable from the persons themselves (p. 315).

Responsive style

Just as 'freedom to learn' opens for the learner both an enticing and a frightening opportunity, so for the facilitator, 'freedom to learn' suggests experimentation, creativity, autonomy, and inevitably, a degree of power. Exercising choice in facilitation has been taken up by Heron (1977) who suggests six dimensions of facilitation with opposite poles.

> Directive–non-directive: Facilitator takes responsibility or delegates the responsibility to the learner.
> Interpretive–non-interpretative: Facilitator gives meaning to activity or indicates behavioural activity.
> Confronting–non-confronting: Facilitator challenges distorted

behaviour supportively or creates a situation for self-confrontation.
Cathartic–non-cathartic: Facilitator actively elicits cathartic release or creates a tension-releasing situation.
Structuring–non-structuring: Facilitator creates process for specific types of experiential learning, or provides experiential learning which requires no structure.
Disclosing–non-disclosing: Facilitator shares own feelings or remains silent.

(Heron 1977, quoted in Beckett and Wall, 1985)

The list implies that the facilitator selects among many styles during one episode with a student. Consider a facilitator who wants the student to be emancipated, and believes in liberation from rigidity and control. Consider another who protects the student, and facilitates by exonerating and covering up for less than satisfactory performance. What underlies the different approaches? Is it possible for clinical teachers to vary their facilitation style to accommodate the situation, the student and their own distinctive personal needs in that episode or occasion?

One could say that pursuing a cognitive outcome of clinical teaching suggests a facilitation that challenges intellectual responses and sets high expectations of theoretical understanding. The power of the cognitive model of nursing has implications for the balance students achieve between cognitive reasoning and affective sensitivity. Clinical teachers who regard an affective outcome as more important, and who aim to decrease the anxiety of students, are probably prepared to accept mitigating circumstances to excuse a less than high standard of performance. The implications are that emancipation, freeing the student from dependence on the teacher, may not occur. Finding the middle ground between a helping and a challenging style may be one of the most demanding tasks in clinical teaching.

No doubt your choices of styles of facilitation will be influenced by several considerations, such as the confidence, or on the other hand, the lack of assurance of a particular group of students, their level of knowledge and skill, their progress in professional development and the ease or difficulty of the clinical assignment.

In considering the different styles of facilitation it may be useful to refer again to the examples of facilitation in a problem-based course as described by MacMillan and Dwyer (1989), where the skill of challenging through questioning is a major component (see

Chapter 4, p. 112). Townsend (1990b) also gives a picture of a facilitator in a problem based course in this example:

> Facilitators work alongside students: to provide support and demystify the learning process; to identify appropriate and necessary resources; and to provide a secure environment in which everyone can experiment, take risks, increase their acceptance for uncertainty and develop mutual trust and commitment. Facilitators are creative, flexible, motivated and involved in mutual goal setting and achievement (p. 67).

Clearly, clinical teachers require a repertoire of facilitation skills sharpened through experience and based on knowledge of individual students and the clinical or community specialty, and applied according to what can only be called their 'clinical teaching wisdom'.

5.5 RESOURCING

One of the most difficult resources to activate is the opportunistic happenings in the environment. The ability to see opportunities and use them distinguishes clinical teachers as persons with ingenuity and flair.

Opportunistic clinical teaching

Activity:
Think of a recent opportunity you have seized and used for teaching. What was it and what did you do? What was the response from students? Ask your colleagues the same questions and compile a set of examples of opportunistic teaching. When you have compiled the examples identify whether the most interesting examples come from acute care areas, from community placements or from nursing homes or other extended care facilities.

Feedback:
The tendency is to think that acute care offers more happenings, but that is not necessarily the case. Opportunistic teaching is not dependent on the ease of availability of interesting or unusual events but on making opportunities for students to learn. Again, very different from the clinical assignment which is tailored in an orderly way to allow for continuity, sequence and integration as required by the curriculum, opportunistic experiences usually emerge as realities unfold.

How does the clinical teacher make use of these opportunities? Even when the opportunities are of an emergency or stressful nature, it is possible to make some preparatory arrangements, for example,

1. negotiating beforehand with the clinical or community staff to take one or two students to assist;
2. immediately follow up to 'debrief' the student to reduce stress, and later, to allow the actual learning to be identified and shared with the whole group.

Opportunities for students to be involved actively with the clinical teacher during, for example, the management of a disturbed elderly person in an otherwise uneventful programme in a day centre, are valuable and to be encouraged. Students will find the experience of reality stressful, but, as reported by Chapman and Chapman (1974) preferable to the unrealistic written 'interpersonal exercises' often used as simulations. They quote students who say that '. . . written analysis of the interpersonal record of what went on between patient and self leaves many students cold', and that it 'primarily forces one to be a certain way on paper with no opportunity to hash out the process realistically. Many of the students frankly relate that they fudge on who said what to whom' (p. 161).

Opportunistic learning as discovery

Working 'blind' with students is not advocated, and it is true that when the clinical teacher is personally acquainted with individual students and 'sensitized to the kinds of behaviour that trigger positively and negatively charged actions and reactions' (Schweer, 1972 p. 54) opportunities can be manipulated to allow individual students to explore, take risks and survive.

One of the surprising, but not infrequent, comments students make in clinical is that they have 'nothing to do'. Underlying the comment is the assumption that 'real' learning best takes place in action-packed high-visibility 'high-tech' environments, where even observing from a distance is a vicarious involvement for students. In low-visibility areas where the pace is slower and the events less dramatic, students often wonder how these experiences contribute to their preparation for competence when their turn comes. Having 'nothing to do' is often another way of saying 'this (event, situation, area) and the people here aren't involving me. Therefore I'm excluded and don't belong. Give me important things to do so that

I'm part of it, or show me how I'm part even though I'm only a learner'.

Opportunistic teaching can use such indications to advantage. One tactic is to use the continuity of concepts across nursing settings and activities to show the interdependence of learning in different settings and practices. Schweer puts it this way: '(continuity) provides sustained and recurrent opportunities for skills to be practised or concepts and skills to be developed from small beginnings into major meaningful concepts and abilities' (Schweer, 1972, p. 108).

What does this mean for opportunistic teaching? Norris's (1975) article 'Restlessness, a nursing phenomenon in search of meaning' gives ideas of the value of tracing restlessness in many aspects of life, and of course, in the variety of forms of restlessness in patients. Involving students in such a project to investigate and understand the phenomenon means that observations can be made 'opportunistically' when occasions arise, for example, when a clinical assignment is cancelled suddenly, or for some reason the clinical programme for that day meets unforeseen contingencies. The continuity is important as the project is not just a 'fill-in' to make the best of an unfortunate change of direction for the day, but is deliberate and part of an on-going project which will eventually trace the different manifestations of restlessness in other settings and areas of practice. Preparation for nursing in areas of acute care where restlessness may be an important sign for expert observations is an obvious purpose of the project. Students can be encouraged to nominate other phenomena for observation and study.

The formal programme of clinical learning represents only a selection of experiences possible for students. Opportunistic teaching can alert students to observations they could otherwise miss. To make full use of unanticipated events which could be observed you need to prepare students in advance by:

1. indicating at the beginning of the clinical module that you will find opportunities for them to observe unusual or unfamiliar events;
2. explaining that each opportunity will involve a specific focus for observation, for example, put themselves into the situation; what would they have done or said; what understanding do they have of the events; what did they observe which was missed by those in the event;
3. pointing out that they will be expected to discuss their observations with the whole group later.

Opportunistic teaching is also important in developing students' observation skills in their direct 'hands-on' activities as well as being a spectator of happenings around them. By taking opportunities to guide students to discriminate, recognize and interpret what they see, feel, smell and 'sense' you can convey a personal interest in their efforts to become 'good observers'. You could use exercises to develop perceptual skills (e.g. figure/ground problems) which help students to explore how their interpretations of what they see are affected by factors such as what they expect to see; want to see; or have been instructed to see (Héath, 1979).

You could also use opportunities to make sure that students learn how to derive meaning from their observations rather than merely being an interesting diversion. Compiling even brief pocket-notes on observations over a period of time helps develop skills in categorizing and sharpening perceptions.

Brief assignments in the form of observations can be used to advantage as opportunistic learning. Requests such as the following may be deceptively casual; in reality they are tied to a well-developed teaching/learning style which engenders discovery:

1. I'll help you work out how to position Mrs Jones to give her some relief, first have a look at what we did for Mrs Thomas, then you tell me what you think the major problem will be, and what we can do about it, then you can show me how we can fix it.
2. I would like you to take a look at the patient you looked after yesterday . . . I think there are some changes . . . see what you think.

Opportunistic teaching is just as important in community placements where observations of everyday activities often seem unnecessary to inexperienced students. It is important that the observation is not a 'spur of the moment' suggestion – 'go and observe the children in the play centre' – but the directions should include what to observe, what to assess, investigate or question, reactions and recommendations. 'Observe the play materials in this child health centre. What criteria guided the choice for this age group? How did the children use the materials? What are your recommendations for change based on your observations?'

If you are sufficiently well acquainted with the setting and the programme of activities and have a few plans ready 'opportunistically' you could also provide an advance organizer, such as suggesting that the student revise the developmental stages of pre-school children and the role of play for this age group. Depending on the level of students you could also suggest an organizational framework the students could use for storing and retrieving the information later (Watts, 1990). The 'opportunistic' observation exercise has the possibility of widening the students' perceptual and interpretive skills and increasing their abilities in linking what is observed with underlying theoretical concepts.

Daily access to resources

The human, administrative and community resources available to a program are usually well mapped out for the faculty and there are also guidelines in texts to suggest how to access and work with resource persons (Infante, 1985), human, administrative and community resources (Schweer, 1972), space, setting, library and multimedia laboratories (Reilly and Oermann, 1985) and contractual agreements with agencies (Carpenito and Duespohl, 1985).

So far we have dealt with what most clinical teachers do and with some of the ways they assist students to learn. In the next sections we will look at what may help and what may hinder teaching and learning in clinical/community settings.

5.6 THE ENVIRONMENT FOR CLINICAL LEARNING AND TEACHING

Assuming that the clinical facility has been chosen for its potential for rich experiences, we shall now look at what influences the learning environment and what the clinical teacher can do to maximize opportunities for learning.

Activity:
Think back to the last week with your students. What were the major influences on you and the students? Were the influences constraining or facilitating? How did you overcome the constraints and maximize the facilitators to make the environment more conducive to clinical learning?

Feedback:

Physical setting

Although individual students and clinical teachers are likely to react differently to the colours, odours, sounds, technology, architecture and locale of the setting, whether institutional or community, it is important to remember that the impact of the physical environment can be strong. This is particularly the case for students whose previous experiences of an affluent and comfortable environment have protected them from the realities of social and economic differences. It is not unknown for students to leave the course because they find the physical setting for clinical practice to be stressful. Turning what is a constraint for some students into a facilitator for learning, is a challenge. What can the clinical teacher do?

Preparation of students for the setting seems essential. Brief visits to observe and identify stressors in the physical environment could be followed by analysis of the impact experienced by individual students. Next, an exploration of the possible effects of the setting on patients can often bring a realization that nursing is not only concerned with one-to-one relationships of nurse and patient, but with interactions between nurse and patient and their immediate environments. Studying the context of clinical practice in a variety of environments and institutions (childrens' units, accident and emergency, extended care, community agencies, and the locality of patients' homes) can bring reality and involvement that television simulations in the lab cannot do.

Geography of the setting

Most clinical teachers are constrained by physical settings where contact with students is spread across several locations. The impact on the clinical programme is immense. If time is not to be spent mostly in travel to and from student placements, a different clinical programme needs to be designed. For example, clinical teaching can be achieved by joint appointments of clinical staff between agency and educational programme; or the development of handbooks and clinical guidelines for students in a self-directed mode. The involvement of the clinical staff is vital so that the students have resource persons at hand.

Social setting

The uncertain, unpredictable and unique environment of clinical teaching is exemplified as much by the social system of the setting as the clinical components. Social, emotional and political dimensions exert influences which operate as constraints and also as facilitators for learning.

Clinical teachers and clinical staff each operate within their respective social systems. Yet, there is clearly a need for the two systems to work together and to overlap in their relationships. For example, negotiating the assistance of expert clinical staff for specific aspects of clinical assignments, and alternatively, accepting requests from the clinical staff to teach a particular topic, require that clinical faculty and clinical experts interact and understand each other's social systems.

The emotional dimension also influences, not infrequently, the participants in the clinical setting. For students and clinical teacher the range of emotions through pain, frustration, fear, helplessness, anger, shame, guilt, as well as joy, wonder and love can be experienced. Sometimes interpersonal conflict arises between patient and student, student and clinical staff or student and clinical teacher. Accepting that there will be clashes of personality from time to time regardless of the skills of the clinical teacher is being realistic. Several reasons, including the physical and emotional health of either party in the relationship could be the underlying factor. Having an understanding of the pressures on students who are learning, studying and practising, as well as coping with developmental stages of their age group may enable the clinical teacher to arrive at a reasonable response and thus avoid a break-down of the relationship. The clinical teacher also has personal needs and responsibility for other students, and clinical time may be too limited to expend on one of the students to the detriment of the others' learning. The resumption of trust could begin with an acknowledgement that the relationship is in difficulty and an arrangement made to discuss the problem later. It is important to make clear that, if necessary, there are opportunities for the student to be transferred to another teacher, without prejudice.

Political policies such as the establishment of contractual arrangements for access to clinical facilities enable clear guidelines to be implemented to secure boundaries and to spell out the roles and responsibilities of clinical staff and faculty. However, when the policies and procedures are resistant to change, the standards, roles and responsibilities may act as constraints on updating clinical practices and learning programmes. Power, status and prestige are part and parcel of the life of an organization. The coercive nature of power in withholding information, expertise and rewards can operate as a vigorous constraint in the clinical setting. On the other hand, collaboration and co-operation are facilitating factors which students should have opportunity to observe and practise.

Professional practitioners in the setting are influential in the students' learning, yet insufficient integration of practitioners into clinical teaching can be responsible for lack of harmony and misunderstanding between health care service goals and the learning goals of the educational program. Powell (1988) examined this problem and found a need for an alternative to the jargon-ridden lengthy curriculum-type directions so often handed out. Assuming that qualified practitioners will be prepared to read, understand and accept the material as guidelines for students is presumptuous. 'Quite naturally then, in busy clinical settings', Powell notes, 'the qualified practitioner becomes more interested in what the students can do rather than what they can learn' (Powell, 1988, p. 72).

Distractions in the setting – competing demands

The richness of the environment is a facilitating factor but the competing demands of the patient's condition and the situation for the student's attention can act as powerful constraints. Students can be distracted from their clinical and learning tasks by the complexities of the clinical environment and the patient's need for care and attention. At times the clinical teacher expects the student's attention while an explanation or a suggestion is given, while at the same time, the student is trying to come to terms with the patient's distress, or with other unsettling events in the immediate vicinity. What can the clinical teacher do?

Your response could involve guiding the student in recognizing priorities to order the steps in the clinical task. You could also select appropriate means and time to give explanations and make suggestions so that the student benefits by being able to concentrate on the major demand at that time.

Time demands

Time constraints also have a critical impact on clinical teaching and learning. Carr (1983) in her observations of clinical teachers and students noted that teachers maintained a certain pace throughout the day so that activities would be completed. 'The pace was fast, busy, constantly in motion, teacher and students interacting whenever they found each other together' (p. 138). The purpose of many of their interactions with students related to time and the language teachers used was punctuated with time-reminders such as 'don't get too far behind' and 'don't forget what time it is' (p. 138).

An interesting exercise for any clinical teacher is to keep a log of the day's activities, over a period, as a way of discovering the impact of time on the demarcation of responsibilities. The log will also indicate how your activities change from the initial days of contact with students new to the area to the last days of their clinical term with you. Carr concluded that time was so influential in the teacher/student relationship that her model of clinical teaching includes 'time-limited process' as one of the primary concepts. Three phases of working within the time limitations were identified in her observations (pp. 345–346): Exploration and uncertainty, where the teacher

> gathered student performance data, compared it with intended purposes, assessed learning styles;
>
> established standards and expectations for performance;
>
> monitored closely;
>
> established a working relationship with the clinical area personnel.

Working, where the teacher

> employed preferred ways of operating to achieve the intended purposes.

Closure, where the teacher

> lessened preferred ways of operating in terms of detail the intensity and student terminated the relationship with celebration activities.

We have isolated only some of the elements in the environment for clinical learning and teaching to identify their constraining and facilitating factors. There are, of course, many other aspects making up the complex environment which affect the learner and the teacher and they have been mentioned in Chapter 1. Continually weighing up the effect of the environment for teaching is important. It is equally important for clinical practice, and as this is the environment in which graduates will practise as qualified professionals, students' attention needs to be lifted, from time to time, to take in the wider context of their clinical assignments.

The next section deals with the selection, design and conduct of clinical assignments.

5.7 CLINICAL ASSIGNMENTS

The views on the purposes of clinical learning change over time and, at present, some of the traditional methods are being challenged for their capacity to reflect the complexity of effective teaching and learning. One of the arguments is whether clinical assignments should be structured or unstructured.

Activity:
In some programmes students are simply assigned to a particular clinic, ward or community agency for their clinical experience. In other programmes a clinical assignment with objectives, information and a certain amount of direction is given to students. In your programme what would be the advantages and disadvantages of (a) the structured and (b) the unstructured, clinical assignment in assisting students to learn?

Feedback:
The design of the students' clinical learning experience will depend on what your faculty has decided are the purposes of the clinical practice session in the program. If your faculty agrees with Infante (1985, p. 128) that '. . . each hour spent by the learner in the clinical laboratory should be devoted to learning, that is, the transfer of theory to practice' the planning of experience will reflect that aim. Additionally, Reilly and Oermann (1985) suggest that the purpose of clinical practice in an educational programme is 'to become skillful in the use of theories of action' (p. 4) and in learning how to learn, how to handle ambiguities, think like a professional and be responsible for their own actions. Taking Benner's view, the clinical setting is always much more complex than the theories learned in the classroom and 'presents many more realities than can be captured by theory alone' (Benner, 1984, p. 36). Carpenito and Duespohl (1985) are definite that the students are in the clinical setting to learn professional nursing and their plans for learning should reflect that aim to prevent their being called upon for 'extraneous non-professional activities'.

At this point it could be helpful to consult your school's statement of philosophy and your programme as a whole to identify what is considered to be the purpose of students' time in clinical or community settings. (You may be surprised to find an explicit statement that has been forgotten, or that changes in thinking have occurred since it was written, or alternatively that there is a bland phrase which defies serious consideration).

Structured clinical assignments in the clinical learning cycle

If your programme uses the cyclical approach to clinical teaching and learning, the clinical practice component has a definite purpose in the students' learning. Following the lab and briefing sessions, students possess sufficient knowledge and skills, and are ready to put their learning into action in the care of the specific patients or clients to whom they have been assigned. Students in their senior years will be assigned several patients, or will have various assignments to mirror the responsibilities they will have later as professional practitioners. They will also have assignments where they will be expected to derive knowledge from their observations, experiences and practice.

The purpose of assignments in the community will be related more to learning to participate in primary health care teams, and to work with communities.

The advantages of structured clinical assignments in the clinical learning cycle are

1. for the student:
   (a) clarity in expectations and standards;
   (b) selected in terms of students' levels of learning and experience;
   (c) benefit of 'advance organizers' in preparation for learning in new and unfamiliar experiences;
2. for the clinical teacher:
   (a) allows written record of experience;
   (b) allows knowledge of readiness and preparedness of students;
3. for the clinical/community staff of the hospital or agency, advance information written especially for staff rather than a copy extracted from a formal curriculum document.

The disadvantages of structured clinical assignments are:

1. could be a straitjacket, holding some students back;
2. the design of the assignment could be boring without interest and diversity;
3. students could be prevented from recognizing experiences other than those contained in the assignment.

Clinical placement with unstructured assignments

In some programmes an extended period of time may be spent in a clinical or community area. Apart from a list of general objectives to be achieved for the period as a whole there may be no further directives.

Some of the difficulties with this format are described by Carlson *et al.* (1987) who advise more explicit written guidelines for students. 'Nurse educators agree on the need for objectives in the classroom situation and frequently communicate them in a written form. Written expectations for clinical, however, are rarely given to student nurses prior to their clinical experience. Clinical expectations are understood by instructors, but communicating them to students results in mixed interpretations' (p. 194).

Other clinical teachers, however, consider that there are advantages in less structured clinical experiences. The advantages and disadvantages of unstructured clinical assignments are summarized below.

1. Advantages:
   (a) freedom to develop an individual approach to practice;
   (b) more suitable for students in senior years;
   (c) provides opportunities to gain from working with clinical staff; to experience the 'real world of work' rather than spending most time on the completion of an assignment;
   (d) opportunity to recognize the scope and limits of responsibility;
   (e) provides occasions to identify individual coping mechanisms in emergencies, unfamiliar, frightening or disturbing experiences;
   (f) allows individual attempts to integrate previously acquired knowledge with current observations.
2. Disadvantages:
   (a) likely to be 'hit and miss';
   (b) students not sure what is expected;
   (c) if unable to identify personal goals, uncertainty about achievements, frustration and disappointment results;
   (d) difficult to identify criteria for credit.

Selecting clinical assignments

Activity:
Imagine that your programme has decided to design structured clinical assignments for students in junior years. Each faculty member is to design assignments for the students in the module for which he/she is responsible. How will you select and design the assignments for your students?

Feedback:
The issue here is how much freedom do you, as the clinical teacher have? In reality, the objectives of some programmes have already determined that a sequence of experiences be undertaken for successful completion of the programme. In other programmes the team of clinical teachers together decide on the assignments to be given to students. If you can select the assignments yourself what guidelines are available to assist you?

First let us look at the experience of some clinical teachers in the USA. McCoin and Jenkins (1988) surveyed clinical teachers and students in 15 nursing programmes in USA and found five ways of selecting student assignments in common use. The methods of assignment were:

1. instructor set (assignment)/student gathered (information);
2. instructor set/instructor gathered;
3. student set;
4. staff set;
5. combination of both.

The preferred method used by the 15 programmes surveyed was the instructor set/student gathered method, although students found some anxiety in gathering information. Among the advantages of the instructor set/student gathered method were:

1. opportunities for students to research:
   (a) medical diagnosis
   (b) nursing interventions
   (c) medications
   (d) principles
   (e) lab test values
2. anticipating nursing diagnosis;
3. learning to read the chart;
4. increasing students' motivation;
5. decreasing student anxiety;
6. assessing the patient;
7. becoming familiar with equipment.

The major disadvantages were:

1. time spent in compiling information for the assignment/(approximately one to one and a quarter hours per assignment);
2. time students spend in commuting, researching and developing a plan of care;

3. cost of travel/distance;
4. difficulty for some students in choosing relevant information;
5. tendency to focus on problems;
6. increase in numbers of students arriving together to read charts, and ask questions.

In comparison with the wealth of information sought about the patient's physical condition (medical diagnosis, surgery (planned or completed), medications, activity level, allergies, diet, special treatment, communication disorders, mental and physical assessment data, safety needs, significant past history, lab data, fluid (intravenous and oral)), information on the cultural, social and religious needs was rated low by students and even lower by faculty. The development of a written outline guiding the collection of information was recommended to overcome some of these omissions.

Understandably, students reported that they were more secure when the clinical teacher made the clinical assignment and gathered the material. It would be expected that the students' quality of preparation for the assignment would be less than if they had met the patient and gathered the material themselves. Because of the amount of time necessary to be spent by the student in compiling information, the question arises of whether credit should be awarded for the work done in preparation. On the surface this seems a reasonable suggestion. On the other hand, the balance of the importance and value of the time spent in planning for the assignment and in the actual experience of doing the assignment would need careful consideration. The deciding factor needs to be the balance between the advantages for the students' learning and the improvement of patient care (McCoin and Jenkins, 1988).

Designing clinical assignments

Based on clinical objectives. Carr (1983, p. 321) describes a method of designing assignments for students by interpreting clinical objectives. The objectives always direct students to do things. The teachers studied by Carr thought about the objectives, gave them a certain value and then used them to assess the most suitable and available clinical learning situations. Teachers chose situations in which the student's needs and the desirable outcomes of the situation could both be met; and lastly, chose objectives which best fitted the learning which would occur in the assignment. Carr comments that in using this method, the clinical teacher revealed the knowledge and skills that he/she most valued. In addition, regardless of the programme goals for clinical teaching 'the teacher's behaviours were guided by their intended purposes for teaching and the educative environments created by each teacher reflected their intended effects on student behaviour. However, the clinical objectives were vital because they provided the general parameters for teacher decision making' (p. 322).

Chase (1983) describes another method of designing clinical assignments:

> Each clinical experience is carefully planned with behavioural objectives for that day or week. The clinical assignments are made the day previous to the experience to enable the student to pre-plan. They have enough information to write patient goals and interventions. The day of the clinical experience, the students make additions to the patient plan, evaluate and change interventions as necessary. The instructor has briefly visited the patients before preconference and can share patient conditions and changes that may have occurred since the assignments were made (p. 348).

Jones (1983) believes that clinical objectives are important in designing assignments as they indicate to the student, instructor and agency staff the level of performance expected and the degree of independence desired for each behaviour. For instance, an objective that states that 'the student will be able to teach patients with diabetes' is not specific enough to indicate what learning experience is needed to meet the objective. A more accurate statement of the objective, Jones suggests, is 'given a patient with adult onset diabetes, the student will be able to teach proper foot care' (p. 256).

Based on community placements. In some programmes the distance between placements prevents the clinical teacher having frequent contact with each student. In this circumstance prepared guides for both teacher and students' use during a unit or module of study can be helpful. An example of a typical guide will have the following content:

1. directions for use of the guide;
2. aim and objectives;
3. questions to be used as a pre-test;
4. timetable;
5. the learning package.

The learning package contains an outline of content with questions. In the case of a problem based programme, the outline will be in the form of a problem situation which will be dealt with in class. In a concept-based programme the outline will show how the major concepts can be identified and understood within a selected group of person-related and situation-related problems. In other programmes the outline is presented in a traditional manner such as a case study or presentation. Both teachers' and students' guides contain the same outline of the content. The teachers' guide also gives suggested teaching strategies. Both guides contain the work required for practice, the method of and criteria for assessment.

Based on students' needs. How often do clinical teachers select clinical assignments according to student needs? In Goldenberg and Iwasiw's (1988) study to identify the criteria for selection of patients for clinical assignments the rank order of criteria was: first, the students' individual learning needs; second, the patient's nursing care needs; third, matching the patient's needs with student's nursing needs.

The authors point out that the method of selection indicated by their respondents does not automatically represent their actual practice. In fact, the lack of evidence of any rationale in selecting patients for individual students gave rise to the study. Of interest in tracing the influences on faculty are the findings indicating that older faculty members 'gave more importance to the student, the nature of the clinical environment, and to themselves than did younger teachers. Increasing age, experience and maturity not only cause concern over workload and health, criteria identified by these respondents, but presumably allow faculty to focus on the student as a learner, to recognize their own influence upon student learning, and to place a high value on the clinical field and staff' (Goldenberg and Iwasiw, 1988, p. 262).

The authors also report that when the ratio of students to teacher is high, teachers have less time to assist students individually and they then rely on the learning resources in the clinical area to provide resources that match the curriculum, rather more than they match the students' needs. The authors' final comment is that the selection of patients should be 'a rational and thoughtful process. Graduate programmes that prepare nurse educators should include in their curricula the process of patient selection and the criteria used to achieve this' (p. 263).

The selection and design of clinical assignments have lasting effects on students' learning. Windsor (1987) reports that students prefer difficult assignments because this shows that the clinical teacher trusts the student and the tough questions help them to learn. Students report that a wide variety of clinical experiences with 'lots of different diseases', 'different kinds of floors' 'a variety of instructors' and 'working with different equipment' all increased learning. Students also reported that the type of assignments given them was important because through well-structured assignments they will learn 'knowledge and skill acquisition, time management, and professional development' (p. 152).

Basing the selection of patients on the students' needs raises a number of questions in relation to the needs of students to meet the requirements of the clinical programme, the needs of students identified by you, as their clinical teacher, and the needs expressed by students themselves.

The individual nature of the needs you and your students identify indicates that a fine discrimination among students should be made to match the students' needs with individual patients' needs. Take, for example, the range of life-style differences between students and patients. How can students learn to develop a system of values if they are protected from experiences which put their values to the test? Students are likely to experience the ethical complexities within life and death issues in emergency or life-threatening diseases but find that on a social and behavioural level their previous experiences are of little guidance. Students may affirm a set of values in principle, but find it difficult to implement those values in actually caring for patients whose preferred way of living is in direct conflict with their own. Reilly (1990) claims that students need their values challenged and asks 'In selecting clients for our students or graduates, how often do we select a client whose values and life-style differ from those of the student or graduate? I suggest that the selection of clients is made primarily on the basis of some illness or developmental criterion, rather than on an affective learning basis reflective of the philosophy of our code and standards' (p. 94).

So far we have looked at the styles and skills of clinical teachers in helping students to learn, the effects of the environment on learning, and the variety of designs of clinical learning assignments. In the next section we will explore how the quality of the clinical experience of students can be nurtured.

5.8 QUALITY OF THE CLINICAL EXPERIENCE

No matter how much clinical exposure students have, the quantity does not necessarily ensure that the experience will promote the students' personal and professional growth. The quality of the experience is related to the opportunities students have for understanding what the experience means and for coming to terms with issues such as life and death, ethical dilemmas, personal responsibility and accountability for one's own actions. Most of these issues are personal and individual but the clinical teacher can assist in ensuring that the students have sufficient experiences of quality to allow them to engage the issues.

We will explore quality under three areas:

1. personal learning needs and personal knowledge;
2. translating personal learning needs into teaching and learning actions;
3. indicators of quality of clinical learning experience.

Personal learning needs and personal knowledge

Activity:
In the briefing session, you encouraged your students to identify their personal learning needs. You did this by giving assurances that there were other things to learn apart from the clinical objectives of the programme, and that these were likely to be aspects known only to them which they could keep private or they could discuss with other students in the group. They agreed to share and came up with the following:

1. I want to be able to understand what's happening here – I keep changing – doubting the things I always believed in.
2. I get pretty distressed sometimes – when there's a death – I don't know where I am with all of it.
3. I want to know how I'm really going – as a nurse, I mean.
4. I wish I knew more – I'm so green.
5. Sometimes I feel great, then bang! I'm right down again – I think I'm scared a lot of the time.

In the clinical/community setting they are expecting you to help them. What experience will you arrange for them?

Feedback:
First let us analyse what you did. In straightforward terms you were really asking them for their 'personal objectives'; they came up

mainly with personal interests and feelings. You assured them they could retain their comments as confidential, or they could reveal themselves to the group. So, you recognized the uniqueness of each individual and the right of personal integrity; you respected each one's worth and their need to know about themselves. When they opted for discussion with their peers they were free to analyse each other's personal needs and to affirm their personal worth. In other words you had set up a way of enabling the group to experiment with 'personal knowledge'. That was fine for the briefing session, but now you are in clinical or community in a predominantly action-oriented environment and you cannot raise students' expectations without following through to assist them.

How will the students' brief excursion into personal knowledge help them? Notable writers in the field of education (Dewey, 1938; Phenix, 1964; Smyth, 1984; Carr and Kemmis, 1986; Schon, 1988) caution against the restrictions on human personality of learning experiences which are predominantly technical and practical and which can lead to little more than depersonalization of the clinical task. In nursing, as in other health professions, educators have a 'responsibility for improving the quality of human meanings at the deepest personal level' (Phenix, 1964, p. 197). Nurses can re-iterate many experiences in clinical where their self-knowledge was challenged and their approaches to patient care were altered. Opportunities to deal with the changing perceptions of themselves and with the meaning of the experiences for their further development were not readily available. Phenix points out very clearly that 'Effective teaching in this domain requires extraordinary insight into the profound depths of the human mind and a level of understanding far different from the judgments of practical life' (p. 348).

Is this beyond the framework of clinical teaching as we know it? Not according to Benner who traces the role of personal knowledge in the development of clinical knowledge in these terms 'As a nurse gains "experience", clinical knowledge that is a hybrid between naive personal knowledge and unrefined theoretical knowledge develops' (Benner, 1984, p. 8). Benner says that the actions and decisions made in clinical are due to a transaction between personal knowledge and the particular clinical situation. Expert clinicians are needed, therefore, to model how they combine their personal knowledge with the clinical situation. We would add that expert teachers are needed who are aware of the value of personal knowledge and who can arrange graduated experiences in clinical situations where students can discover the source of their developing clinical knowledge.

Is this beyond the abilities of the clinical learner? Not according to the students who are continually questioning the meaning of health and illness and their own developing insights. Much depends on the individual clinical teacher to realize that 'Learners including neophyte nurses cannot help relating new learning to past experiences. By doing this they bring their own personal meaning to the learning situation and thus make learning a combination of the information itself and their feelings about it . . . Each person brings his own particular history, intellectual commitments, and readiness to learn to a particular clinical situation' (Benner, 1984). The philosopher and educator Phillip Phenix claims in *Realms of Meaning* (1964) that 'in personal insight the simplest and most untutored people can be as competent as, or even more competent than, people who have devoted much time and thought to the perfecting of this aspect of life' (p. 196).

Is it beyond the objectives of the clinical educational programme? Not according to Lindeman who believes that it is clear that packaging clinical experiences in the 'nice neat boxes' of the traditional approach does not match the demands of the everyday realities of clinical learning and teaching. Moreover, Lindeman questions the use of the problem-solving nursing process 'made rigorous by incorporating scientifically derived knowledge' as a model for practice. As such it 'reflects an inadequate understanding of practice, of the knowledge required in practice, and of the dynamic relationship between knowing and doing. Yet this conception of practice is the basis for the organization and evaluation of many, if not most, entry-level programs' (Lindeman, 1989a, p. 27).

There are many clinical teachers who would agree that experience in clinical practice provides more than opportunities to apply sciences taught in the classroom. Acquiring an art of clinical practice is as much a concern of learning as applying theory (Schon, 1988). The art and science of nursing have been the fundamental tenets of nursing practice throughout the ages, so, implicitly if not explicitly, the concept of 'artistry' is at the heart of the clinical program. The problem for the clinical programme at present is not the concept of personal knowledge as a form of the art of nursing, but the balance of emphasis given to artistry and science in clinical practice.

Listening to students, it is clear that they struggle to retain their early motivation of caring in a helping profession and at the same time try to master the mounting weight of knowledge and skills expected of them as they progress towards becoming practising professionals. Encouraging expression of their personal interests and personal objectives in clinical learning is therefore a way of providing an outlet for individual aspirations.

Translating personal learning needs into teacher/learning actions

Activity:
Let us return to the student's comments. How will you translate their personal learning needs into teaching/learning actions?

Feedback:
There are several possible options. In the briefing session you would have recognized the stressful nature of the exercise for some students and have taken steps to allay their anxiety. In clinical practice it is important to emphasize that learning the craft and the artistry and developing personal knowledge is not as 'time-related' as the activities in a clinical day. In fact, becoming a clinical expert is a life-time journey regardless of the clinical specialty or whether illness, health or community development is the focus of practice. Putting the students' comments into a time-context is the first step.

Next, the traditional way of selecting teaching/learning actions is to begin with objectives, which have been based on student needs, among other things. Does that format fit your clinical teaching problem? The answer is, yes-and-no.

You could work with the students to clarify their expectations of how they want you to help them. If they request that you be present for specific parts of their clinical assignment, you could work out together what exactly you were to observe or how you were to participate in practice with them. For example, the students who want 'to know how I'm going, as a nurse' would be helped by clarifying what this means. What ideal do they have; how realistic; to be fostered or to be tempered? One occasion of practice is scarcely sufficient as the basis for feedback on such a wide issue. So, working together, a plan could be made for students to see a number of role models and to compare their 'ideal' model with reality, and then identify where, in their own practice they could achieve their personal development and personal knowledge. This is the 'joint experimentation' type of coaching recommended by Schon (1988) as preferable to what he sees as the 'technical rationality' of much professional education.

The 'coaching' relationship certainly offers creative possibilities of working with individual students. If we take the 'follow me' dimension he advocates, your practical knowledge and your own personal knowledge can be used in fine-tuning your guidance. Take, for example, the students who reveal their distress when a patient dies. This reaction is personal, understandable and entirely appropriate. 'I don't know where I am – I'm all over the place' is the occasional disorganized approach you have noticed previously and which now is given a framework by the students, but which they need to understand. They could be helped to see that rather than 'running from the scene', their defence is directionless activity. Coaching students to realize there are other ways of reacting could happen this way:

> Mr Jones' doctor is going to tell him today the results of his biopsy. He's your patient isn't he? We'll stay with him for a while, then we'll talk about it when you're ready.

Coaching rather than teaching (going through the history of the disease, causes, clinical manifestations, prognosis, the possible reactions of the patient, the rights of patients for information and what nursing care to plan) is more appropriate here. The problem is not a lack of knowledge of the patient's condition, but an impending distressing event when he will receive information of life-threatening dimensions. This particular student has indicated that involvement in distressing happenings affects her/his ability to continue to work effectively for some time afterwards. Allowing some time beforehand for the student to anticipate her/his reactions and for you to disclose your possible reactions, encourages freedom and openness and gives permission for feelings and emotions to be acknowledged. The clinical teacher, as coach, remains close, listening and 'feeling through' with the student and the patient from their point of view while taking part in the care, comfort or treatment and guiding the patient and the student.

Your discussion with the student later enables reflection on how you and the student performed with the patient, the implications for the student's immediate activities and the possible coaching needed. Similar to facilitation, coaching can assist students to observe, reflect, interpret and construct meaning out of confusing and puzzling situations. As the coach, you are helping the student in much more than working out how to meet her/his problem. You have shown confidence in the student's capability, a willingness to recognize ideas and suggestions, and the intention to accept the student's plans. Finally, working together with the student leading, demonstrates your willingness to let the student discover her/his own resources of building personal knowledge.

Indications of the quality of clinical learning experience

Most programmes have developed guidelines for the selection of clinical agencies and facilities for placement of students. Criteria relating to setting, staff, clients, and resources are given in Reilly and Oermann (1985) with a specimen instrument for assessment of the clinical setting in relation to the goals of the programme. If the practice of techniques and skills were the sum total of the activities of students' learning we could have confidence in the capacity of carefully selected placements to provide appropriate practical experience. As a mirror of the world of work students will eventually inhabit, the clinical milieu is a fertile ground for personal growth and professional socialization. Once the setting has been selected and placements for students have been arranged, how can we appraise the experience of students while they are in the placement?

Activity:
What indicators have you used to judge the quality of the students' experiences?

Feedback:
We could say that only the students are capable of judging the value of the experience since they are the ones having the experience. However, an authority on experience and education, John Dewey, claimed certain criteria of experience need to be met before the experience can be said to be educational. There should be continuity between experiences and they should promote curiosity, and strengthen initiative. The onus for ensuring the criteria are met falls on the teacher who should be knowledgeable in shaping from the surroundings the experiences that lead to growth (p. 40).

The two concepts Dewey believed to be essential for educational experiences are continuity and integration. Continuity through an 'experiential continuum' leads each experience on to another, for example, 'every experience should do something to prepare a person for later experiences of a deeper and more expansive quality.

That is the very meaning of growth, continuity, reconstruction of experience' (p. 47).

What does this mean for clinical teaching? The quality of the experience depends on widening students' capacity to take on new experiences and to grasp the meaning each experience has for them in the present, and how it will prepare them for future experiences. This involves the clinical teacher in discriminating between worthwhile and less worthwhile experiences and will require directing students towards specific experiences. Take the example of an inexperienced student's first (and unwilling) attempts in confronting an aggressive relative who wants to take a patient out of hospital. The experience allows the student to draw on resources previously untapped, to realize strengths and weaknesses, and to prepare for the next occasion of testing, whether it be in ordinary life experiences or within the professional nursing environment. The continuity of experience would be met by arranging for the student to encounter other experiences where skills could be sharpened and deeper meanings extracted.

This example also shows that experience occurs, not in a vacuum, but in interacting with the surroundings and with others in the environment. The implication is that, as Dewey said, 'experience does not simply go on inside a person' (p. 39).

Important for clinical teaching is Dewey's claim that 'There are sources outside an individual which give rise to experience. It is constantly fed from these springs' (p. 39). Again, the clinical teacher is active in searching for experiences which will extend students' growth and self-knowledge.

It is in the debriefing session in the clinical learning cycle where students and teacher can reflect on and pursue the meaning for them of each experience. This will be effective only to the extent that the clinical practice has included experiences of quality.

The extract below is from John Dewey's *Experience and Education*. Take some time to read it and to reflect on its implications for discriminating among worthwhile and not so worthwhile clinical experiences.

> The belief that all genuine education comes about through experience does not mean that all experiences are genuinely or equally educative. Experience and education cannot be directly equated to each other. For some experiences are mis-educative. Any experience may be such as to engender callousness; it may produce lack of sensitivity and of responsiveness. Then the

> possibility of having richer experience may increase a person's automatic skill in a particular direction and yet tend to land him in a groove or rut; the effect again is to narrow the field of further experience. An experience may be immediately enjoyable and yet promote the formation of a slack and careless attitude; this attitude then operates to modify the quality of subsequent experiences so as to prevent a person from getting out of them what they have to give. Again, experiences may be so disconnected from one another that, while each is agreeable or exciting in itself, they are not linked cumulatively to one another. Energy is then dissipated and a person becomes scatterbrained. Each experience may be lively, vivid, and 'interesting' and yet their disconnectedness may artificially generate dispersive, disintegrated, centrifugal habits. The consequence of formation of such habits is inability to control future experiences. They are then taken, just as they come. Under such circumstances, it is idle to talk of self-control. Traditional education offers a plethora of examples of experiences of the kinds just mentioned (Dewey, 1938, p. 25).

5.9 ROLES OF THE CLINICAL TEACHER WITH STUDENTS IN THE CLINICAL/COMMUNITY SETTING

Activity:
It is time to go back to the previous stages of the clinical learning cycle, the lab and briefing sessions, to recall the clinical teachers' roles in those sessions. Which roles do you consider are also appropriate for you in the clinical/community setting? Which ones would you omit, and which additional roles do you suggest?

Feedback:
After scanning the roles we have identified so far, you may consider that most of the roles are appropriate for teaching in the real setting as well as the simulated lab or briefing. Certainly the teaching/learning roles such as facilitator, coach, supporter, challenger, helper, resource person and colleague apply. The roles related to organization, planner, manager and co-ordinator also apply as do the professional roles such as researcher, inquirer, professional role model and expert clinician roles.

While it is true that the clinical teacher has a role as an assessor of students' clinical performance we have not included that aspect of teaching/learning in this chapter. Instead, the *feedback* role has taken its place as a specific teaching/learning strategy with the emphasis on informed guidance towards improvement.

We acknowledge the problem of role conflict when students perceive a contradiction between the teacher as facilitator and supporter and at the same time as assessor responsible for contributing to decisions which could influence the students' progress in the course as well as threaten their self-esteem. Creating a learning environment conducive to the clinical teacher as assessor centres on development of mutual trust and respect.

The specialized subject of assessment and evaluation of clinical performance is beyond the scope of this text. The views on the purposes of clinical learning change over time, and as ideas and expectations are sharpened, it is clear that the traditional methods of assessment of clinical performance are limited in their capacity to reflect the complexity of effective clinical performance and learning. The evaluation of clinical performance remains an area of challenge awaiting manageable solutions.

What additional roles are there for the clinical teacher? The role as *observer* comes into its own in the clinical/community setting and needs to be added as an important role, ongoing and integral to the assessment of the impact of the environment on learning and to the ability to give specific feedback to students and to helping them interpret what they see around them.

The *learner* role of the clinical teacher occurs implicitly throughout the clinical learning cycle through the many opportunities of observing how students learn, and through the continual inquiry into and search for knowledge. In the clinical/community setting the focus of the clinical teacher includes learning with the student how to develop clinical knowledge, recognize researchable problems, and raise issues for theory development. Importantly, learning about one's own performance and gaining insights into self-knowledge is at the centre of being a learner in clinical/community practice.

Closely related to the learner role is the role of *co-experiencer*, centering significantly in the experiences of students and patients. The role requires clinical knowledge, familiarity with the students' progress in learning and the patients' response to health, illness and prognosis. You will probably recognize the close relationship of the coach role as you consider the step by step involvement as a co-experiencer in the life events of students and patients.

Finally, the role of *carer* underpins the clinical teacher's activities in clinical practice. The nurture of students, commenced in lab and briefing sessions continues and extends into the full caring role as an educator, with students and patients. At its best the caring role is unobtrusive, almost hidden, but is evident in the careful selection of learning experiences in the interests of students and patients, in the warm empathic presence and in the intuitive concern for the welfare and growth of students, patients and self.

6

Debriefing: reflecting on practice

6.1 INTRODUCTION

Debriefing of students and the clinical teacher after clinical practice is the focus of this chapter (Figure 6.1). Debriefing is not the end of a cycle of learning and practice, rather it leads once again into briefing, clinical practice and debriefing.

Recent thinking about experience-based learning has broadened the concept of the 'post-conference' in nursing education and shifted the emphasis from recounting events in a clinical assignment to analysis of the students' experience itself. Debriefing has been accepted in Australian nursing as a more appropriate way of capturing what the student experienced as well as what was done, and then to extract meaning and learning from it.

How much of the clinical day should be spent in debriefing? Is it necessary to debrief students every day or only at the end of a clinical/community placement? What kind of teaching/learning session is most effective for debriefing the students' experiences? Would there be advantages in combining several groups of students and clinical teachers from different practice sites in a debriefing session?

This chapter aims to explore the challenges of debriefing for both the clinical teacher and students, to explore perspectives on the purposes of debriefing, to suggest alternatives for conducting the sessions, and to identify the implications for clinical learning and clinical practice.

By the end of this chapter you will have identified the purposes of debriefing in the clinical learning cycle, explored a range of approaches to debriefing, determined the clinical teaching skills

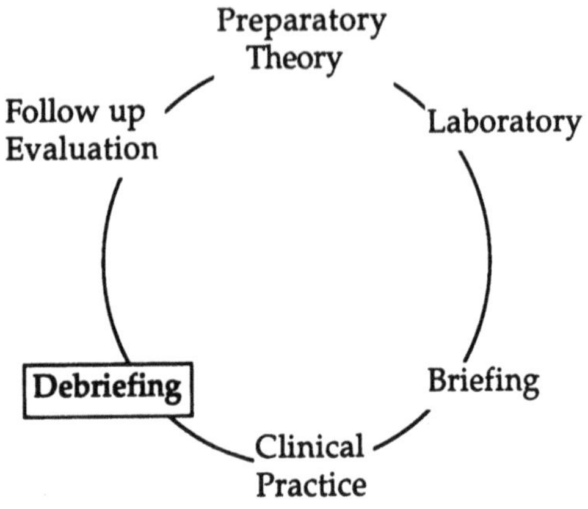

Figure 6.1 Clinical learning cycle: debriefing.

and reviewed the roles of clinical teachers in debriefing and in the clinical learning cycle.

6.2 PURPOSES OF DEBRIEFING

Activity:
Imagine that you have been asked to justify to your institution the inclusion of debriefing in your module. You have decided that the purposes of debriefing are not sufficiently understood and should be made explicit. What will be included in your purposes and how will you address this problem?

Feedback:
You could structure your justification by explaining

1. your responsibilities for students' performance in clinical practice in accountability, ethical and cost-benefit terms;
2. your educational responsibilities in assisting students to develop nursing skills and to learn that professional nursing practice is subject to scrutiny and analysis.

Purposes related to responsibilities for students' performance

Debriefing is a follow-up of the students' performance to see whether clinical objectives had been met. Debriefing can also address accountability for the standard of the students' and your own performance. Professional self-examination ('wherein the supervisor would have his or her work subjected to a rigorous analysis similar to the analysis of the (student's) work') was advocated by Goldhammer (1969, cited by Retallick in Smyth, 1986, p. 92).

Ethical issues related to the patient's/client's rights to safety, privacy, confidentiality and information and the students' rights to appropriate clinical education can be examined in a debriefing session. Matheney (1969) also included the development of generalizations and guidelines in providing nursing care and keeping the focus on 'patients as people'.

A cycle of learning which enables preparation, practice and review is cost effective in that it makes the most of costly clinical placements. Debriefing is a significant component of the cycle where feedback is given to students on practices to be corrected and improvements to be implemented.

Purposes related to educational responsibilities

The purposes of debriefing are directly linked to the learning, clinical assignment and experience foreshadowed in briefing and transacted in practice. The purposes therefore include:

1. *Learning*: estimating progress in personal learning and knowledge;
2. *Clinical assignment*: giving and receiving feedback on the conduct of the assignment;
3. *Experience*: 'turning experience into learning' by analysis of the clinical experience, structuring reflection and deriving meaning from the experience (Boud *et al.*, 1985).

You may have selected for your justification of debriefing, purposes that are more relevant to your programme, the level and stage of students' learning and your own personal philosophy of clinical teaching. In respect of purposes related to your programme's goals you may share with Matheney (1969) the view that debriefing enables clarification of relationships between theory and practice or with Lindeman (1989) that deriving theory from experience and practice is a more appropriate statement of purpose.

You may have linked some purposes to particular educational goals such as group sharing of clinical experiences and problem-solving (Reilly and Oermann, 1985) or instead, problem-posing and helping the learners to become students of their own work (Smyth, 1984, 1986).

Although we began the purposes of debriefing with a justification in management terms, we do not mean to give priority to those issues above others, but rather to keep a realistic approach to the contextual structure in which clinical teaching and learning exists and in which health care, management and education are partners.

You may have noticed a progression from the older to more recent purposes of debriefing. That is not to say that the positions of Matheney (1969) in nurse education or Goldhammer (1969) in teacher education are inappropriate today, but rather, to observe that the emphasis on reflective processes has changed the nature of the debriefing session.

Let us try to trace these changes from our understanding of the purposes of debriefing. We could say that debriefing has evolved from a semi-formal session where the purposes were for the clinical teacher to help students in group problem-solving, analysis of practice, exploration of theory and practice, clarification of thinking and feeling to less formal, more interactive sessions characterized by purposes such as giving and receiving feedback, exchanging meanings and interpretations of the experience in a collegial relationship of students and teacher. The current trend in debriefing sessions is the inclusion of purposeful reflection in learning how to learn from experience.

For further reading on purposes of debriefing see the following nurse educators: Matheney (1969); Burnard (1987); White *et al.* (1988(a)); Lindeman (1989(a)); and teacher educators: Goldhammer (1969); Turney *et al.* (1982); Smyth (1984, 1986); Boud *et al.* (1985); Boud (1988); Pearson and Smith (1985).

6.3 PREPARING FOR DEBRIEFING

Is it necessary to have a plan, or should the discussion be unstructured and simply take a lead from the spontaneity and pace of the students? We take the view that any learning session needs a plan which will meet the session's purposes, is flexible and able to respond to students' needs.

This section includes:

1. planning the programme of sessions;
2. implementing the plan;
3. organizing the sessions.

Planning the programme

Activity:

You have decided that although debriefing in this phase of the session focuses on the students' clinical experience you are going to try to work out a programme which will give some structure and direction to the debriefing sessions. What guidelines will you use in constructing the programme?

Feedback:
Debriefing the students requires small problem-solving groups and individual one-to-one sessions for feedback on performance. Debriefing the students' experience requires structured, purposeful reflective processes.

Setting the objectives. These can be derived from the purposes. For example, debriefing the students suggests objectives related to 'group sharing of clinical experiences'. Remember that the preparation for learning in the briefing session included addressing the students' concerns and personal learning needs. Objectives related to those issues are just as important and, for some students, more so. Debriefing the students' experience suggests objectives related to 'analysing clinical experiences' by 'structuring reflection' and 'determining future behaviour or practices'. The clinical assignment is part of the experience and objectives related to the performance of the assignment need to be included. Students need feedback on their performance, their progress in self-directed learning and other negotiated practice. Objectives to guide the feedback process are required.

Sequencing. It may be desirable to sequence the sessions from less demanding and complex clinical assignments to ones more inclusive of a range of clinical skills by the end of the module. It is important that such sequencing is explicit and that students have a sense of how the debriefing sessions are planned to develop their clinical learning.

Selection of the experiences of students as the focus for the sessions. This is a consideration if you are going to debrief the students after every clinical day. Does every student's experience need to be included at each session? An alternative to allow for realistic timing of each session is to select a focus (for example a clinical practice or learning problem requiring management) that has emerged during clinical practice and is agreed by the students to be significant. This allows flexibility and also enables the sequencing of the sessions to be related to the students' increasing knowledge and skills.

Teaching/learning strategies for the debriefing sessions. It is important that debriefing retains a vitality throughout the module so that students come with an expectation that the session will hold interest and significance on top of what they have experienced in clinical practice. There will be some group problem-solving (or better still posing problems about nursing actions, or interventions so that taken-for-granted routines are challenged) and there will be one-to-one feedback with individual students at the conclusion of the session. Having a wide repertoire of skills and strategies is as essential in debriefing as it is in any other teacher–student encounter.

Identifying student outcomes. This is not so appropriate for this session. In fact, specifying outcomes is the major difference between debriefing and the previous stages of the clinical learning cycle. Each student's experience is known only to that person, understanding its meaning will have a different outcome for each individual. Certainly outcomes such as the intentions of students to revise, or further develop skills, knowledge and attitudes can be stated, but again these can best be identified by the student not the teacher.

Review and evaluation of each session. This needs to be included in the plan as a joint exercise for students and teacher. It is important to establish whether students are gaining what they expect and need from the sessions so that they can proceed to the next stage in their clinical practice placement.

Implementing the programme. The process of planning a programme of debriefing sessions appears to be no different from any other teaching/learning programme. There are, however, important differences in the implementation of the plan.

If you want the session to link the students' experiences with the topics of your module you have two options. You could select a topic for each session so that students can know ahead of time what the substantive topic will be. Your teaching/learning strategy will include deriving from clinical practice those principles you intend that students should grasp in relation to the topic. For example, you could identify issues relating to bioethics associated with the clinical experience, and then use those to exemplify your topic. The obvious difficulty with that approach highlights the alternative option. Why not have a list of topics you intend to include in debriefing, and which are known to students, but leave the choice of topic for a particular session so that it can be linked more directly with experiences most students have had that day? The value of 'opportunistic' learning could then be appreciated by students. In addition deriving meaning from practice as it occurs has advantages over the first method which could become contrived and more subject-related than experience-generated.

In focusing on practice, students' behaviour and experiences, many clinical teachers would see a difficulty in progressing from student to student to ask for their report. At the same time, it should be said that debriefing is not merely an invitation to students to 'rehash' what they did, and to receive comment on how well or badly and what to do about it. So, many teachers would claim that it is better to choose a topic, from the theoretical programme, which is relevant to the clinical area, and lead a discussion around that topic. We take the view that, although linking theory with practice is to be encouraged, to focus on a subject or a topic is more appropriate for a tutorial before clinical practice than debriefing after the experience. As Cox (1990) notes, 'the subject matter is already integrated within the patient and clinical practice, only its separation is artificial'. He raises a question which is important for focusing on the students' experience: 'How can the questions of practice be assisted by theory?' (p. 566). Posing problems which arise directly from experience uncovers previously unchallenged assumptions for examination.

Certainly, students might ask for an explanation of an observation they have made, or you might need to correct a misunderstanding about a physiological process or a misinterpretation of a behavioural manifestation, and therefore reference to theoretical content is required. The focus is the observations and experience of practice made by students and described in their own clinical language. The focus is not a description of a text-book case with accompanying formal language. Your usual interactive style of questioning or facilitating can show to students that from their experience, they themselves can often untangle the parts of a clinical observation to make sense of a confusing picture.

Organizing the session

If you want to draw from each session the meaning of experiences for each individual student, and also the development of new ideas for clinical practice that all the group can use, you will need to keep the group together. (There are several models of focusing on experiences in the group which are included later in the chapter.) Giving and receiving feedback, if not already part of clinical practice, can occur in a session with individual students. Allowing sufficient time for debriefing is essential. One hour seems to be the absolute minimum to allow for the two phases (beginning with debriefing students, followed by debriefing of experiences).

The considerations outlined for organizing the briefing sessions apply to debriefing also. The location of the session adjacent to the clinical or community placement is an advantage for contact with resources, or with clinical/community staff. Again, as in briefing, the inclusion of the relevant resource persons or clinical/community staff for selected periods of the session is desirable, more for a full appreciation of the students' experience than for evaluation of performance. Feedback from the clinical staff could be given later in a three-way feedback session of clinical teacher, student and clinician, if there are to be gains for all three participants.

6.4 CONDUCTING THE DEBRIEFING SESSION

Many clinical teachers would agree that a debriefing session is one of the most difficult sessions to conduct. By considering debriefing in two stages, both the needs of individual students and their experience can be managed in the session.

Debriefing the students

Students at the end of a clinical day often present a range of reactions. Stunned disbelief at a clinical emergency and its sequel of frenetic action and perhaps tragedy and death; excitement at being involved in a rewarding clinical experience; frustration that nothing seemed to 'go right'; exhaustion from tension or from physical activity starting with a late arrival, no breakfast and trying to catch up all day; anger overflowing from a conflict with the clinical staff; delight at a series of pleasant experiences and performance which resulted in praise from the clinical staff. Add to that another range of feelings not yet disclosed and also your own reactions to the clinical day. You now have a group very different from the anxious, tentative and anticipatory group you prepared in the briefing session. The individual students you coached, guided, supported and observed in clinical are now here as a group again.

Activity:
Would it not be better for them to relax and then come back to debrief? What kind of session will this be? What will guide your behaviour with this group in debriefing?

Feedback:
Although you and the students may be fatigued, and possibly at times stressed, debriefing as soon as possible following practice while the experience is fresh has several advantages. Releasing pent-up feelings within the group of peers and a sensitive teacher is more desirable, and healthier, than 'sounding off' to others who do not know the context or the experiences. For feedback to be effective it is important that it be given as soon after the events as possible.

Debriefing is one of the few occasions in nurse education where the focus is the student's own behaviour and experience. Whether the theoretical programme is problem-based, concept-based, competency-based or follows a particular nursing model, in the classroom or lecture hall the focus of the students' learning is the content of the subject even though the student (or problem, clinical condition or community situation) and styles of learning may well be a major consideration. In the lab the context is the simulation of events or problems, through which basic principles are tested and where skills are mastered through practice. Briefing prepares students (and patients) for a set of specific clinical/community experiences, clinical practice structures the assignment and experiences with patients, families or communities, but in debriefing the focus of the students' learning is the students, their behaviour and their experiences.

If we accept that view of debriefing there is little need to state the obvious, namely, that it is not another typical group discussion or individual encounter, and that guiding your behaviour will be the knowledge that the students (and yourself) are not the same persons as when you met together in briefing. Whether their clinical experiences are perceived as positive or negative, they have reacted and responded with behaviour that now needs to be recalled, analysed and understood. The experiences for many have been completely new, often unpredictable, and frequently unexpected.

Also guiding your behaviour is the knowledge that individual students need to debrief substantive knowledge and skills to use in their next cycle of clinical learning. You are also aware that it will be difficult for students to learn if they are carrying over from clinical practice their anxieties and concerns. In the early writing on debriefing (post-conference) Matheney (1969) gives this advice:

> Certain ground rules govern the conduct of postconference. One of these is that affective experiences with strong student reaction take precedence over anything else, whether related

> to the learning focus of the day or not. As long as students are preoccupied with strong emotional reactions, no learning will take place anyway until the feelings have been ventilated or resolved. Frequently students' emotional reactions serve as take-offs for a valuable learning experience (Matheney, 1969, p. 288).

The colleagueship between you and the students established in briefing and clinical practice is even more appropriate in debriefing. The focus is on the students first, and then on their practice. The advantages of being with the same groups of students is, of course, that you have a fairly close knowledge of their progress, their characteristic reactions and their developing styles of learning and practice. As you have worked with them both as a co-experiencer and as an observer you will be aware of 'peaks and troughs' in individual student's practice. This knowledge is invaluable in sharpening your perceptions of the student's vulnerability, defensiveness or self-assurance. In fact, you may already have debriefed some students during clinical practice as they questioned 'why did I say that to that patient?' or 'I want to understand what makes me react angrily' or 'I don't know why I'm worried about what I've done because it's really O.K.'. As students begin to raise questions in order to better understand themselves in new situations it is a step closer to their taking a critical approach to confronting their own behaviour. Recognizing the importance of such a step in the student's growth toward critical self-knowing, debriefing 'on the spot' in a one-to-one relationship is to take advantage of a creative teaching and learning opportunity. Health care and nursing in particular, need practitioners who have acquired skills of critical self-reflection.

Your options for commencing the debriefing session have been outlined based on the guiding principle of centring on students' behaviour. You have commenced in an environment of interest and support and in a small group discussion characterized by friendliness and guidance (Rogers, 1969).

6.5 DEBRIEFING THE STUDENTS' EXPERIENCES

This section includes the following:

1. group problem-solving;
2. linking learning, clinical assignment and experience;
3. identifying approaches: technical, practical, emancipatory;

4. reflecting on experience;
5. giving and receiving feedback.

Group problem-solving

If debriefing were simply a reporting back after clinical practice there would be little purpose in students coming together as a group. Each student could be 'signed off' individually at the end of the clinical practice period. Instead they have been prepared to expect that you will help them analyse their experiences and extract meaning from the events and their behaviour. There will also be some group needs. Peer support and group problem-solving could assist some students who have similar clinical experiences and concerns.

What are your options? Perhaps a quick 'round' of all students so they can relate what is important to them? A supportive invitation 'Do you want to tell us what happened to you today?' Alternatively, a period of silence? Or, to start off, a brief run down of your own experiences for their comments? Usually, however, it is better to take a lead from the situation itself. Given the close relationship you have with them it is highly likely that the students will continue to talk amongst themselves rather than regard your presence as a signal that this is a class about to start with a presentation. Then, as part of the group, you could take one of the students' comments as a starting point. Students who have made an outstanding and significant observation, a practical innovation in caring or a perceptive insight into a problem during clinical/community practice may not realize how commendable their particular practice has been. They can be invited ahead of time to tell in the debriefing group what happened and what they did. This is an effective way to commence as it leads into the students' thinking about their practice and into trying to extract meaning from it.

In problem-based programmes students are familiar with group problem-solving, not only in debriefing after experience but throughout the programme. If a problem-based learning programme is successful, students will have learned to analyse clinical problems early in the course and will also have adopted a self-evaluative learning style for their clinical practice as well as their problem-based theoretical studies. Following clinical practice, students could meet in a leaderless group to debrief one another's experiences, seeking the clinical teacher's assistance as necessary.

The suggestion of 'problematizing' as a process – posing problems about the students' practice or the clinical experience, rather than seeing everything as problems to be solved – increases students' ability to challenge assumptions and habit ridden practices (Smyth, 1986).

Linking learning, clinical assignment and experience

Activity:
Having in mind the links between briefing and debriefing let us return to the purposes outlined in the briefing session for preparation of students for clinical practice. Remember, you intended that they would be able to learn, to carry out a clinical assignment and to engage in an experience. How will you and the students find out whether these purposes were achieved?

Feedback:
All through our discussions of the clinical learning cycle you will have noted the impact of the uncertain, unpredictable and uncontrollable clinical milieu on student learning and practice. We could take each component – learning, clinical assignment and experience – and process each one in turn in an orderly sequence. That would hardly make sense. Although the students have been prepared for each separate component, now they have experienced them not separately, but as a whole experience, in environments which are usually not controllable and certainly are changeable. Taking each one separately may appear logically sound, but it does not mirror the reality of clinical practice.

We can easily fall into the trap of reducing clinical experience into elements to make analysis easier and, of course, controllable. But we are trying to find out what students learned through everything that they experienced while in clinical/community. The experience includes personal learning, learning through the clinical/community assignment and learning through experiences. We are also trying to understand what the experience has meant to the students in the group.

Benner (1982a) claims that there needs to be 'a dialogue between what is found in practice, or in the practical situation, and what is expected' (p. 11). That is to say, Benner is concerned that nurses come to clinical situations with the notion that the theory they have learned will match their experiences. The reverse is often the case, as experiences will indicate how practical knowledge can build theory. Therefore it is important that we help students to review what they expected from their past learning and preparation for practice, and what they actually found. Benner claims that clinical situations 'do not qualify as experience' (p. 11) unless such an examination is required. Debriefing provides the opportunity for this exploration.

Identifying approaches

Activity:
Think of the last time you and the students met in a debriefing session to reflect on the recent clinical/community experience. Take a few minutes to think about the approach you used. Then determine which (if any) of the descriptions below resemble your debriefing session.

Feedback:
It is helpful to take time to review the foundations for your clinical teaching. This is particularly useful if your pattern of teaching has been influenced in the past by institutional priorities, a heavy teaching load and an overcrowded programme with little opportunity for personal input or influence.

1. If, in your debriefing, a topic or a problem which students had come across in clinical practice was selected for discussion, the focus of the debriefing session would be decided. That is, the problem or topic would be the central concern and the students would use resources (notes, textbooks, graphs and charts) to review and discuss it. Deciding how to manage it, cope with it and control it would be an expected outcome of the session and a set of guidelines for future practice. You could conclude that the students were prepared for their next briefing and clinical practice, knowing how to deal with that particular problem or topic.
2. On the other hand, if you and the students conferred together about a patient, a family, a community to 'pool' your experiences and to share different observations the debriefing would have a very different focus. The students would be encouraged to include an exploration of the social and environmental influences on the patient (family or community) and on themselves in order to interact with and understand the situation better rather than to control it. You could conclude that the outcome for the students was improvement in their awareness of the context of their patient's or client's practice and a com-

mitment to improving skills in assessing the impact of the social and environmental influences.

3. Lastly, you may have included in debriefing a stage when you and the students considered whether there were any constraints of tradition, outmoded ritual or 'nursing habits' that could stand in the way of innovations. As students and teacher question the validity of some of the theoretical positions that have dictated practice in the past they are empowered to seek within their experience of practice the elements for 'building theory, not just using it' (Lindeman, 1989(a)).

You may have recognized in those hypothetical cameos descriptions of the types of performance associated with (a) technical, (b) practical and (c) emancipatory practices (Carr and Kemmis, 1986; Hedin, 1988). Of course, it is likely that elements of all three approaches will be present in debriefing sessions as they build upon each other. The important point is that preparing students for professional practice includes more than mastery of sets of skills and text-book knowledge. Building personal knowledge out of experience depends on practice in deriving meaning out of experience. Using judgement to discriminate between valuable and worthless experience enables outmoded systems and routines to be challenged. This preparation for professional practice fosters autonomy and critical self-reflection, and creates an atmosphere of empowerment where patients' and clients' participation is sought and encouraged.

Without reflection on experiences, many insights into personal strengths and knowledge remain unrecognized and opportunities for even richer experiences are lost.

The next section explores how reflection can be structured during debriefing.

Reflecting on experience

While it is true that on a purely informal and every-day level we learn from our experiences, on a professional practice level a more informed, intentional and deliberative activity is needed which will direct the way we continue to extract meaning from what we do, think and feel.

Activity:

You have opted for a debriefing session which aims to centre on the students' experiences and your experience with them and to 'turn the experiences into learning'. What will be involved for you and the students?

Feedback:
As more attention is paid to experience-based learning, clinical teachers are searching for a framework which not only explains how students learn from experience but shows how to use experience to achieve learning and changes in behaviour and nursing practice (Boud *et al.*, 1985; Hedin, 1988).

First let us explore the reflective approaches we could use in debriefing. Posner suggests that field experience is captured by the equation

Experience + Reflection = Growth

He adds 'we do not actually learn from experience as much as we learn from reflecting on experience' (Posner, 1985, p. 19). As we saw in the clinical practice component some reflection occurs during practice as students question their perceptions and their activities. In fact, according to Schon it is the reflective practitioners who are freed from the constraints of tradition-bound thinking and are able to create alternatives. On the other hand, without reflection, practitioners are more likely to follow, uncritically, familiar routines and traditions than to search an experience for new ideas or to work out and test alternative strategies.

Let us take an example, using the personal needs expressed by students and incorporated by the clinical teacher into coaching these students. What can reflection in debriefing achieve? Remember the student who asked 'I want to know how I'm going, as a nurse'? During clinical practice (Chapter 5) there were opportunities fostered for the student to reflect-in-action on what she/he meant and activities were arranged so that the student could observe a number of role models as a basis for identifying what approach she/he wished to take. During clarification it became clear that the student's question was related to the conflict caused by the image of the nurse who comforts and the one who must at times cause pain (e.g. during painful dressings or procedures).

Through reflection with the clinical teacher's and the group's help the student could return to those experiences 'turning a subject over in the mind and giving it serious and consecutive consideration' (Dewey quoted by Posner, 1985, p. 19). It is important that judgements are reserved at this stage so that the experience is recaptured entirely according to the individual's perspective. A set of questions can be used (privately or within the group) to analyse what happened, for example:

1. What did I expect to notice in the roles of experienced practitioners?
2. What did I actually notice?
3. What surprised, delighted, disappointed or confused me?
4. What did I discover, and what can I infer from the discovery?
5. Where do I now stand in relation to my own perceptions of my role as a nurse?
6. What does this mean for me? Will this work for me if I take it on board?
7. What will the costs be for me if I decide to try this?

Activity:
Let us look at the model for reflection in experience-based learning proposed by Burnard (1987). This model has five stages:

1. practical experience;
2. sharing of experience;
3. reflection in a group, on that experience;
4. discussion based on the outcome of reflection – new learning is planned and developed;
5. evaluation of learning and planning to apply the learning.

How would you use Burnard's model to assist your student to 'turn experience into learning'?

Feedback:
It is helpful to have a model as a guide for the reflective process. In order for the debriefing session to assist students to derive meaning from their experiences the session needs careful planning to avoid a simplistic 'talk-back' session. Burnard explains his model in these terms:

> Essentially, the students develop practical experience in the wards or community. When they come back into the school, they reflect on that experience. Then, in stage four of the cycle they decide upon their learning needs out of that reflective period. At this stage, the tutor may also offer suggestions as to how they may proceed, based on the tutor's knowledge of the syllabus and the nursing curriculum. At stage five, learning is evaluated and preparation made to apply the new learning in the clinical situation. The students then return to the ward, or

community, to use the new learning and the cycle begins again (Burnard, 1987, p. 192).

Burnard draws attention to the need for the clinical teacher to consider the individual student's unique personal experience and at the same time to draw the group together to extract shared meaning from the session which all members can apply to the next clinical experience. The cycle of events in this model fits well with the clinical learning cycle and its use could demonstrate to students an experience–reflection–new experience process which assists both learning and practice.

You could use this model to plan the sharing of experiences in stage three above. Students in small groups could tell each other their experiences, returning to the large group to share with the clinical teacher the group's comments on common experiences and the learning needs identified. Individual experiences, different from the group, could also be brought into the large group so that all students are involved and receive assistance from the resources of the whole group.

Stage five of Burnard's model suggests the inclusion of feedback and evaluation of learning. The clinical teacher's input is necessary to carry over observations of students' performance made in clinical practice. This would be especially important for those students who had asked for specific areas of their practice to be observed and also for those who negotiated contracts for self-directed learning.

Activity:
You may still be concerned about how to manage the reflective process in debriefing. Have a look at the model for 'turning experience into learning' (Figure 6.2). Can you apply the steps to the questions the student is asking of herself during reflection?

Return to experience. The student in Figure 6.2 did this. (Reflection is a form of response of the learner to experience.)

Attending to feelings. It is possible that this occurred during the initial 'debriefing the student' phase of the session. (Using positive feelings, removing negative feelings.)

Re-evaluating the experience

1. *Association.* The clinical teacher is aware of and sensitive to the nature of the student's experience through the opportunities

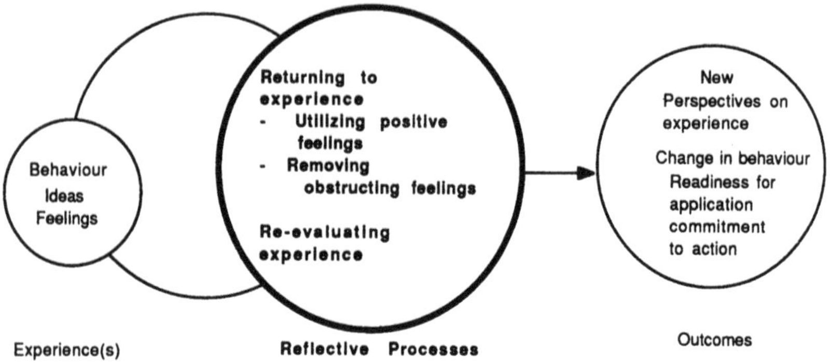

Figure 6.2 How to help students learn from experience.

Source: Boud (1988).

provided in clinical and can now assist the student in relating new ideas and information to previous relevant attitudes and knowledge. (Observing how RNs interweave comfort with painful treatments; noting the superior technical skill which minimizes pain for the patient; discussing with RNs and patients their feelings following an episode of treatment.)

2. *Integration*. The student's question about discoveries, and inferences could lead to insights which can then be taken into and meshed with the ideas the student is developing. (Developing an understanding of perception of pain in self and the pain of others; exploring contexts which increase or diminish pain; developing skills in recognizing signs of impending pain.)
3. *Validation*. The questions asking 'What does it mean for *me*; is it real?' could involve a 'try-out' in the reality of practice. (Adopting a different or new awareness of the practice role in which an ability to see pain as unavoidable at times in healing, while at the same time retaining sensitivity to the reality of pain in another and compassion in caring.)
4. *Appropriation*. Accepting the new approaches and understanding into one's own value system involves answering the question 'Will this work for me if I take it on board?' (Changing one's view of self is involved as well as the values associated with self as nurse.)

Debriefing is an ideal time for assisting students in deciding on the changes in practice, behaviour and learning which they want to incorporate into their experiences and to specify what actions they plan to take. There are obvious links here with feedback on individuals' performance.

Boud's model suggests that readiness for a new experience follows reflection. However, the benefits gained from reflection could be merely an exercise in abstract thinking if the experience is not linked with future actions.

While it is true that clinical experiences are amenable to learning by simple reflection both during and following the experience, it should be noted that every debriefing session need not be wedded to the above schedule of reflective processes. Critical reflectivity can be demanding for both students and clinical teacher in the beginning of a module when the participants are new to the clinical setting or community placement. When students and teacher have had several clinical experiences together, reflection on those experiences can be facilitated by the colleagueship and co-operation in the group as well as by the knowledge and interest of the clinical teacher.

Giving and receiving feedback

Students' performance in clinical practice. The clinical assignments which have been part of the students' experience are important episodes of practice (provided that they have been selected appropriately as outlined in Chapter 5). During clinical practice the teacher, observing students' performance and noting important aspects for special comment is able to choose appropriate ways to communicate this information to students. For both the clinical teacher and students this is an important learning time.

How will the teacher communicate the observations made:

1. In measurement terms, indicating from objective data, the number of correct and incorrect actions according to criteria which have been set by the programme? (This may be appropriate for learning skills for safety of practice where each element must be mastered. Such learning is practised and mastered in the lab.)
2. In nursing process terms, tracing the steps in problem identification and nursing diagnosis according to the way the nursing plan has been designed, conducted and reported? (If changes have occurred making the plan less relevant, will the process of making the changes and adjustments, and the basis for making those judgements be included in the feedback?)

3. In terms of telling (giving the 'evidence') or in assisting students in interpreting the actions or behaviour? (Sergiovanni (1986) suggests that feedback as 'food for thought' rather than 'evidence' captures the fullness of what actually happened in practice. Since the context of complexities and uncertainties is the daily environment of clinical practice, a feedback approach which considers performance against this moving background seems to be required.)

Importantly, the following suggestion for feedback in teacher education can also apply to nurse education. The student is portrayed as a human information processor who

> interacts with the evidence, interprets its meaning, decides its relevance, and determines whether and how it will influence his or her thinking and subsequent decisions. In other words, the purpose of evaluation of information is to promote informed intuition. Informed intuition enables supervisor and teacher to reflect on their practice with greater understanding, to enhance their collective professional judgment and to make better decisions about this practice (Sergiovanni, 1986, p. 49).

Turning back to debriefing the student's experience according to the Boud *et al.* (1988) model, the debriefing process enabled the student, with the clinical teacher's and the group's support, to engage in similar information processing. The student arrived at an interpretation of the meaning of the experience and followed this by identifying ways to introduce new approaches for trial.

It is important to note that some programmes incorporate feedback which allows a processing of information about performance so that the teacher can indicate where the performance requires improvement and the student can indicate plans for when and how the practice will be improved. The responsibility is on the teacher for providing concrete and specific feedback and on the student for contracting the methods taken to attain improvement and the standard to be achieved.

Self-evaluation

First, there will be individual needs as some students have opted for self-directed learning in clinical and others contracted with you for certain clinical experiences. Others have individual 'opportunistic' experiences they may want to raise for discussion and review of their response and performance. Still others may simply want to relate what they found, perhaps to their surprise, disturbed, angered, pleased or embarrassed them and to ask for your help in interpretation. There is not much point, however, in rehashing what students have done in clinical, nor in simply having a chat about what they liked or did not like.

As we noted previously it is preferable that observations made in clinical practice are descriptive rather than evaluative, students then have the opportunity of matching their perceptions of performance with yours. There is no need to comment on every performance in detail. Depending on your planning for the program of debriefing sessions, you could choose to offer feedback on those particular performances that illustrate or demonstrate your purposes for that session.

As mentioned in Chapter 5, evaluation of the performance of students, although important, is not within the scope of this text. Evaluation is a programme wide activity in which the criteria, standard and format of evaluations is usually decided. Every clinical teacher requires evaluation skills although all might not necessarily be involved in constructing tests, scales and measurements. Indeed, your programme might have opted for an improvement oriented evaluation as outlined briefly above.

Improvement of performance through feedback as a significant clinical teaching skill is the emphasis chosen in this text. In this context the suggestion of an evaluation portfolio, as a collection of 'life in clinical' makes interesting possibilities.

> Like the artist who prepares a portfolio of her or his work to reflect a point of view, the [student] can prepare a similar representation of her or his work. Together, supervisor and [student] can use the collected artifacts to identify key issues, to identify the dimensions of the [student's practice], as testimony that targets have been met, and as a vehicle for identifying serendipitous but worthwhile outcomes of [nursing] (Sergiovanni, 1986, in Smyth, 1986, p. 48).

Feedback to the clinical teacher

Learning to give as well as receive feedback is an important professional skill to include in the students' experience. Some students choose contracts for clinical practice which required feedback on their performance but also, provide for feedback to be given to the clinical teacher. If you have been successful in building a genuine colleague relationship the interaction can be guided sensitively so that what the student really wants to tell you is actually what is said. An effective contract spells out the behaviour to be performed in advance and these guidelines facilitate the feedback process. It is the nature of clinical practice, however, that unexpected happenings result in unpredictable behaviour. Guiding the student to centre on what was said and what was done before making an evaluative statement about the clinical teacher's performance assists the student in identifying the focus for feedback and assists the clinical teacher in receiving truthful and valid comment on his/her teaching.

As Karuhije (1986) notes, 'Clinical teaching makes two quite different demands on the nurse educator: 1) competence in nursing; and 2) competence in teaching' (p. 142). From whom can the clinical teacher receive feedback if it is not from the students she/he interacts most closely with in these two functions? The aim of a professional interactive feedback process between clinical teacher and students is the welfare of the patient being served and the betterment of the learning of the students being debriefed.

6.6 ROLES OF THE CLINICAL TEACHER IN THE DEBRIEFING SESSION

Activity:

Review the purposes we identified for debriefing at the beginning of this chapter and the processes involved in conducting a debriefing session. What stands out for you as your major roles in debriefing students and their experience?

Feedback:

Your professional responsibilities for preparing students as practising, caring, professional nurses has probably highlighted your *feedback* role. In the lab this role was included in the *colleague* role and the more formal *assessor* role. In clinical practice the emphasis was on improvement through giving informed guidance as the clinical teacher observed the students' performance. In clinical practice the *learner* role included learning about your own performance, and in debriefing there are obvious and important links with the extended feedback role which includes both receiving and giving feedback.

The role of *reflective participant* will, no doubt, be high among your priorities. The role includes *colleague, coach* and *facilitator* but adds other dimensions. In coaching students to turn over in their minds the events in their practice, you have reflected with them on their 'blind spots', helping them to see themselves at work as nurses and interpreting with them their behaviour from their point of view, and what it may mean. There are similarities with the *learner* role as it is certain that in reflecting with students, you are both extending in self-confrontation and self-knowledge. Finally, there are strong links with the *professional role model*. Where personal learning, interpretations and meanings are entrusted in the teaching/learning relationship it is important that reciprocal standards of ethical personal behaviour, of confidentiality and discretion are maintained.

6.7 CONCLUDING COMMENTS ON THE CLINICAL LEARNING CYCLE AND THE CLINICAL TEACHER

As we mentioned in an earlier chapter, some programmes include a 'total course debriefing' at the conclusion of a module or unit of learning where students, clinical teachers, course staff and clinical staff come together to hear from each other how the programme actually worked. For example, how appropriate was the selection of content of the theoretical component and the method of teaching for assisting transfer to clinical problems? Could there be a closer link of the lab programme with the key theoretical concepts and principles students are expected to master as the foundation for learning skills for practice later in the clinical context of patients' problems? How effective were briefing sessions in preparing students specifically for clinical learning, clinical assignments and clinical experiences? In particular, was the selection of clinical placements and experiences conducive to clinical learning and, finally, were the debriefing sessions able to achieve their potential for raising insights into practice and learning, and introducing commitment to changes in practice and behaviour?

The results of the review can lead to important changes, or at least modifications, to the programme, the teaching, or the selection of placements, and the cycle begins all over again. We commend the practice of 'total course' debriefing because of its value in reviewing the sequential nature of clinical teaching and learning throughout the cycle and the mechanisms for integrating content and the strategies of clinical teaching. We also acknowledge however, the difficulties of allocating sufficient time and the logistics of arranging meetings of participants from across several institutions.

Sometimes, a framework such as the clinical learning cyle becomes a mere strategy or technique which develops a life of its own, and is followed slavishly. Reviewing its effect on the participants is a responsibility of the clinical teacher in the role of *educator* and *researcher*. Research on the clinical learning cycle and its implications for learning and clinical/community practice is essential. Self-examination by several clinical teachers could reveal interesting differences and could give rise to innovations. Student opinion should be sought not only through each stage of the cycle, but preferably, on the cycle as a whole unit. It is not until students have been through several cycles of briefing–clinical practice–debriefing that the effect of such an approach for their own practice style can be evaluated.

Introducing the cycle for the first time, or perhaps introducing innovations to traditional clinical teaching is not a short-term exercise. As *action researcher* the clinical teacher can plan, introduce and act, monitor, review and replan through each stage of the clinical learning cycle.

In the clinical teacher's role as *educator* and *leader*, the clinical teacher can take the initiative to introduce workshops, in-service programs and courses for the education of clinical teachers. The quality of clinical education has direct effects on patient/client/community care and student understanding, caring practice and personal growth. As we saw in the first chapter, the assumption that almost anyone can teach in clinical settings if they have classroom teaching experience is wrong. Clinical teaching is a specialized field requiring of its practitioners knowledge, skill acquisition and personal care and commitment.

The further development of clinical teaching as a field of study and practice will require recognition of its academic importance and extension of its theoretical foundations.

7

From student to nurse

The previous chapters in this book have described the components of a cycle which represents a phased process of clinical teaching and learning. Representation of such a complex phenomenon in such a way is, of course, simplistic but it helps us to analyse the various parts of the teacher's task and to question and improve some of those practices which we have long taken for granted. This chapter fills in the background to the clinical teacher's task. It considers the context and culture of clinical teaching and the process of becoming a nurse. The clinical nurse educator is, above all, the colleague who is most responsible for initiating the novice to his or her profession. To do so without an appreciation of the subtleties of that process would be to miss the most potent opportunities available for shaping the future practice of nursing.

7.1 BECOMING A NURSE

The process of becoming a nurse is a social one. It should be distinguished from the academic process of earning a degree or qualification. The latter process signifies that the individual has the required attitudes, skills and knowledge to practise competently. In contrast, professional socialization is the process by which the individual learns the culture of nursing: that combination of symbols, customs and shared meanings which makes nursing distinctive. Many nursing academics are involved in the elusive pursuit of a description of that culture – it finds expression in the multitude of theories of nursing or 'philosophies' of nursing which form the introductory section of all nursing curricula. By its very nature, however, culture is hidden, it is implicit in what is done, it is reflected in the unconscious but shared assumptions of its practitioners.

Nursing is an evolving culture which is being redefined constantly by its practitioners and by changes in health systems and needs. While not denying the importance of recording philosophies and theories which will guide that redefinition it is nevertheless important to recognize that immersion in the culture 'as it is lived' rather than as it is seen by 'armchair theorists' is an important part of learning to be a nurse. This carries an inherent risk of conservatism if it is interpreted as a tendency to train students to maintain the status quo but that should not necessarily be the case. The responsibility for encouraging development rather than stasis rests with the clinical teacher who, if she or he is aware of the possibilities, can educate students to reflect critically on current practice and analyse it in terms of its symbolic as well as its clinical content.

The ideal outcome of such a socialization process is a self-image which permits feelings of personal adequacy, satisfaction and autonomy in the interpretation and performance of the expected role. This is, of course, a tall order and may not be achieved by many of our students until they are experienced nurses of some years' standing. Nevertheless, a good clinical education will better prepare them for that eventual outcome.

It must be emphasized that socialization in the sense described above is not about producing stereotypic nurses stamped from a single mould. That is indoctrination, not socialization. The major difference between the two is the extent to which the characteristics of individuals are permitted to influence the outcome.

Socialization is a specialized social interaction in which students and the people with whom they come in contact develop expectations of themselves and each other in the clinical context and respond to each other with those expectations in mind. It goes without saying that this will only occur if students find themselves in real clinical situations with reasonable frequency and with realistic roles to play. Eventually, responses develop into patterns of behaviour and ways of perceiving situations which accord with society's and the profession's views of the nursing role. The important aspect of this process which deserves emphasis is that students themselves have an active part in the process. They are not blank pages waiting to be imprinted with a professional persona. Students bring their own personalities, dispositions and past experiences to the interaction and they should be encouraged to draw on those individual differences in interpreting and responding to the situations they face in clinical. This suggestion may raise insecurities for clinical teachers and clinicians who were trained in a system which emphasized uniformity and standardized procedures but it is an inescapable and necessary consequence of the 'professionalization of nursing'. The future development of the profession and what it can offer the community depends very much on nurturing the creativity and individuality of its new members.

7.2 HOW DOES SOCIALIZATION OCCUR?

A large proportion of the messages students receive is carried in the 'hidden curriculum', those messages both verbal and non-verbal which are conveyed by nurses, patients, doctors, institutional rules and norms. The messages may be parallel with, or may even conflict with, the formal explicit curriculum. This is a particularly significant problem for a profession such as nursing which is undergoing a process of evolution. Practices and norms which are observed in hospital wards, for example, may run contrary to the theories which are being espoused in the curriculum. How should a teacher deal with this when it happens? One possibility is to be critical of outmoded practices or the ignorance of nursing and medical colleagues; another is to try to protect students from such realities; yet another, and more productive, option is to use it as a learning experience, an opportunity to help students develop that critical reflective capacity which will characterize their growing professionalism. This implies the need to allow sufficient opportunity in clinical practice and debriefing sessions for discussion of such 'philosophical' issues. It also means that students should be sufficiently comfortable with their colleagues and teachers to feel free to raise for discussion such apparent contradictions between theory and practice. The clinical teacher could encourage frank discussion by putting the issue 'on the agenda' of the group or by referring to instances which he or she has experienced personally.

Interactions with teachers and nursing colleagues are important socializing influences but are sometimes confusing for students who receive conflicting messages from 'academic' clinicians and clinicians who see themselves as representing the 'real world'. Kramer (1974) described a process of reality shock in graduate nurses who, on entering the world of work, discovered that their nursing-school-bred values conflicted with work-world values. Simpson (1979) described a similar phenomenon. Resolution of this conflict, which is still common in nurse education, will come about only when clinical teaching is fully integrated with clinical work and when all nurses regard themselves, potentially at least, as clinical teachers. Melia (1984) has described an example of the segmentation of nursing education in the British system and concludes that students learn 'neither the education nor the service segment's version of nursing, rather they learn to recognise when one version is appropriate and the other not and fit in accordingly'. She concludes that this practice supports a transient approach to nursing work itself and a lack of commitment to nursing as an occupation.

The existing sub-division of the profession into teachers or practitioners which is reinforced, in Australia at least, by industrial awards, is a significant barrier to the development of clinical nursing as both a field of academic endeavour and as a training ground for professionals. Benner, in her discussion of the stages of development of skilled clinical knowledge, makes the point that nurses at different points in their careers will be at different levels of skill, and advocates planned discourse among nurses at those different levels as a deliberate approach to the systematic study of practice and the development of both staff and clinical knowledge. Similarly, planned discourse between clinicians, clinical teachers and students should contribute to the professional development of all groups. Benner describes a number of strategies for this planned discourse. Innovative strategies include small group interviews in which critical incidents are described in narrative form – narrative language rather than abbreviated synopsis of a case is preferred because it encourages a description not only of the incident but also the intentions, thinking and feelings which accompanied it and which illuminate the 'meaning' of nursing work. Another suggestion is collecting 'paradigm cases' – cases in which the clinical lesson stands out in bold relief. Paradigm cases or cautionary tales (as they have been described in medical education by Ewan, 1985) are a necessary substitute for lived experience but have power even in the retelling because they describe an incident which actually happened rather than framing clinical lessons in hypothetical terms. A third suggested method is to keep records or chart areas in which students and experienced nurses report difficulties consistently. It is probable that these areas are the very ones which require nurses to exercise skilled judgement. Identifying these areas helps the teacher to know where to concentrate effort and helps the student to recognize those areas in which they would gain most from systematically comparing their judgements with the judgements of experts.

Interaction among students themselves is also a major socializing influence. Large scale studies of student culture in the new nursing curricula do not yet exist but the conclusions reached in a seminal study of professional socialization in medicine 30 years ago (Becker and Geer, 1958) are likely to be still broadly applicable to nursing and other professions. Becker and Geer reported the emergence of a student culture which provided a perspective from which students could accommodate to the requirements of the academic programme while directing their efforts along routes other than those suggested by faculty if that appeared to be the most expedient option. Students actively select options for behaviour by balancing personal goals and needs with staff and school requirements. For example, students may be more comfortable maintaining a 'student role' rather than adopting the more threatening 'trainee professional' or colleague role which has been suggested throughout this book. In the student role they may accord priority to book learning and formal classes, devoting less energy and commitment to clinical placements and experience. This type of behaviour will be reinforced if cognitive rather than skill-based and experiential material forms the basis for the majority of assessments. In such an assessment environment the prevailing student culture sanctions postponement of professional role-taking and encourages theoretical rather than reflective learning.

The interactive nature of socialization then becomes apparent – students respond to the most pressing perceived demands of faculty *vis-à-vis* their need to pass examinations. In turn, faculty may complain that students only want to know how to pass exams. The process is circular and self-perpetuating. Melia's work with nurses cited earlier in this chapter also illustrates this aspect of the student culture in action. The culture of the student group and its interaction with faculty should be therefore an acknowledged ingredient in all clinical teaching. Clinical teaching should aim to foster among students an orientation to a professional rather than a 'student' culture where the former is characterized by education as a process of integrating experience and the latter by education as stepwise acquisition of static chunks of knowledge and skill. The social value of the culture of the student group is that it allows students to be flexible and responsive to the immediate needs of their environment. It is the teacher's job to ensure that the environment will encourage the type of professional development that philosophies of nursing espouse.

7.3 WHAT ARE THE IMPLICATIONS FOR THE CLINICAL TEACHER?

The most important implication is that clinical teachers must become aware of the subtleties of interaction which influence the socialization process. Students have the capacity to influence teachers' behaviour as well as be influenced by it. For example, teachers may have to resist the pressure to deliver mini-lectures in clinical or to provide answers in problem-solving group sessions. Students' expectations in this regard are a result of experiences in which previous or current teachers have provided information with students adopting the passive recipient role. These habits are hard to break.

The interactive aspect can, however, be exploited to encourage the development of the colleague relationship among students and between students and teachers. The aim of those relationships should be to share knowledge and experiences and to develop mutual respect and progressive responsibility. Although teachers are unquestionably more experienced as clinicians many of the problems encountered in a clinical context may have more to do with life experiences than clinical knowledge and students may, by virtue of their personal and family experience, have more to contribute in some areas than teachers. Mutuality is therefore possible as well as desirable.

The other major implication is that teachers must re-examine their understanding of their function as role models. Teachers may see their responsibility as being to simply provide a good example for students to follow. Expecting students passively to absorb and incorporate professional values and behaviour patterns, however, is no more appropriate than expecting them passively to absorb the contents of a textbook on nursing theory. Students must be active in experiencing, discussing and evaluating professional behaviour in order to extract personal meaning which can be incorporated into their own self-image. Observing a good role model may help students to understand what is expected of them, but it will not necessarily help them to integrate the forces influencing their own behaviour to produce the desired result. Some students manage to do so but many experience some form of strain in accommodating to their professional roles. Part of that strain results from the fact that the achievement of technical competence does not ensure the ability to perform as a competent professional and clinical teaching often fails to recognize those parts of professional competence which are not encompassed by technical and cognitive mastery of clinical tasks.

One potential pitfall to avoid is the tendency to concentrate on the technical 'training' of students and to miss the opportunity to foster their personal growth, self-conception and psychosocial resources. This tendency results from the ease with which technical criteria can be defined by faculty in contrast with criteria for personal development of students. It also reflects the tendency to view technical competence as the public face of education while personal development is the private face and not perceived as the responsibility of the curriculum or the teacher. If 'thinking' and 'doing' are separated from 'feeling' and 'being' the curriculum and the learning environment assume a scientific and technological culture which inhibits expression of feelings and reflection on those aspects of experience which complement technical competence. This problem has long been recognized in medical schools in which the scientific/technical culture and context results in the observation that 'the teacher must remain unaware of what is happening to the student. The defences freeze into rituals in which teacher and learner alike shut out the human voices of the patient and the doctor in distress' (Marinker, 1974). Clinical teachers can, if they are aware of the need, avoid this becoming true also of nursing curricula.

7.4 WHAT CAN THE TEACHER DO?

Teachers can provide consistent opportunities for taking the professional role in a supportive environment with respected senior colleagues who are sensitive to the processes of socialization and who could provide insightful, constructive feedback. Teachers can assist professional development by making the hidden curriculum explicit; by revealing not only the cognitive aspects of clinical reasoning but the intuitive and affective aspects as well; by exploring the implications of alternative clinical actions not just from the clinical viewpoint but from the viewpoints of professional, patient and society (Good and Delvecchio Good, 1980; Stein, 1984). Teachers can help students to develop a healthy perspective on professional responsibilities by exploring stressful situations and the variety of responses exhibited by other students and by experienced nurses. Teachers can, by broadening the repertoire of venues for clinical learning, also contribute to the students' experiences of the realities of clinical practice in a variety of contexts which do not provide the technical and psycho-social support services found in teaching hospitals.

In summary, clinical teachers can recognize that becoming a nurse is a process of personal development which requires time and space for reflection on experience. Previous generations of students may have fared better in this respect than recent and forthcoming generations who are subject to increasing pressure of content and specialization in curricula. Reflection is a legitimate and necessary aspect of professional education but crowded curricula render it impossible. Curriculum planners and teachers must review the objectives and processes of clinical education to ensure that opportunities for reflection and personal development re-emerge.

Bibliography

REFERENCES

Aggleton, P., Allen, M. and Montgomery, S. (1987) Developing a system for the continuous assessment of practical nursing skills. *Nurse Education Today*, **7**, 158–64.

Andersen, B. (1989) Problem based learning in nursing education: justified or a response to fashion. Paper presented to Education Department, School of Medicine, Southern Illinois University, Springfield, Illinois, November.

Andersen, B. (1990a) An experience in transfer and transformation in nursing education: from hospital schools to the higher education sector. Paper presented to Oxford Polytechnic and Institute of Nursing Studies, Ratcliffe Infirmary, Oxford, UK, March.

Andersen, B. (1990b) The case for learner-managed learning in health professionals' education. Paper presented at 1st International Learner Managed Learning Conference, London, April.

Ausubel, D.P. (1960) Use of advance organizers in the learning and retention of meaningful verbal material. *Journal of Educational Psychology*, **51**, 267–72.

Ausubel, D.P. (1963) *The Psychology of Meaningful Verbal Learning*. Grune and Stratton. New York.

Barrows, H.S. (1984) A specific problem-based, self-directed learning method designed to teach medical problem-solving skills, and enhance knowledge retention and recall, in Schmidt, H.G. and de Volder, M.L. (eds) *Tutorials in Problem-Based Learning. New Directions for Training in the Health Professions*. Masstricht. Van Gorcum, Assen.

Barrows, H.S. (1988) *The Tutorial Process*, Southern Illinois University, School of Medicine, Springfield IL.

Becker, H. and Geer, B. (1958) Student culture in medical school. *Harvard Education Review*, **28**, 70–80.

Beckett, C. and Wall, M. (1985) Role of the clinical facilitator. *Nurse Education Today*, **5**, 259–62.

Bendall, E. (1977) The future of British nurse education. *Journal of Advanced Nursing*, **2**(2), 121–81.

Benner, P. (1982) From novice to expert. *American Journal of Nursing*, March, 402–7.

Benner, P. (1984) *From Novice to Expert: Excellence and Power in Clinical Practice*. Addison-Wesley, Menlo Park, CA.

Benner, P. (1989) Performance expectations of new graduates. Paper presented to AACCN Invitational Conference, Critical Care Nursing at the Baccalaureate Level. Strategies for the Future.

Benner, P. and Wrubel, J. (1982a) Skilled clinical knowledge: the value of perceptual awareness. Part 1. *The Journal of Nursing Administration*, May, 11–14.

Benner, P. and Wrubel, J. (1982b) Skilled clinical knowledge: the value of perceptual awareness. Part 2. *The Journal of Nursing Administration*, June, 28–33.

Benner, P. and Wrubel, J. (1989) *The Primacy of Caring. Stress and Coping in Health and Illness*, Addison-Wesley, Menlo Park, CA.

Block, J.H. (1971) *Mastery Learning: Theory and Practice*, Holt, Rinehart and Winston, New York.

Bouchard, J. and Steels, M. (1980) Contract Learning: the experience of two nursing schools, *The Canadian Nurse*, **76**(1), 44–8.

Boud, D. *et al.*, (ed.) (1985) *Problem-based Learning in Education for the Professions*. Higher Education Research and Development Society of Australia (HERDSA), Sydney.

Boud, D. (1988) How to help students learn from experience, in Cox, K.R. and Ewan, C.E. *The Medical Teacher*, Churchill Livingstone, London.

Boud, D., Keogh, R. and Walker, D. (1985) *Reflection: Turning experience into learning*, Kogan Page, London.

Bruner, J. (1966) *Toward a Theory of Instruction*, Harvard University Press, Cambridge, MA.

Burnard, P. (1987) Towards an epistemological basis for experiential learning in nurse education. *Journal of Advanced Nursing*, **12**, 189–93.

Cameron, S. (1989) Competencies for registration of nurses in Australia, in Gray, G. and Pratt, R. (eds) *Issues in Australian Nursing 2*, Churchill Livingstone, Melbourne.

Carlson, D.S., Lubiejewski, M.A. and Polaski, A. (1987) Communicating leveled clinical expectations to nursing students. *Journal of Nursing Education*, **26**(5), 194–6.

Carpenito, L.J. and Duespohl, T.A. (1985) *A Guide for Effective Clinical Instruction*, 2nd ed., Aspen, Rockville.

Carr, A.M. (1983) Towards a theory of clinical teaching in nursing. Unpublished Doctoral Dissertation, Boston University, School of Education.

Carr, W. and Kemmis, S. (1986) *Becoming Critical: Knowing Through Action Research*. Deakin University Press. Geelong.

Chapman, J. and Chapman, H. (1975) *Behaviour and Health Care*. C.V. Mosby, St Louis.

Chase, B.M. (1983) Clinical experiences made easy! *Journal of Nursing Education*, **22**(8), 347–8.

Chinn, P. and Jacobs, M. (1983) *Theory and Nursing. A Systematic Approach*, C.V. Mosby, St Louis.

Chuaprapaisilp, A. (1989) Improving learning from experience through the conduct of pre- and post-clinical conference: action research in nursing education in Thailand. Unpublished Doctoral Thesis, School of Medical Education, University of New South Wales.

Cook, J.W. and Hill, P.M. (1985) The impact of successful laboratory system on the teaching of nursing skills. *Journal of Nursing Education*, **24**(8), 344–6.

Cottier, L. (1986) Nurse education and Australian studies. Project report. CRASTE Paper No. 14, December.

Cox, K.R. (1990) Learning within practice. *The Medical Journal of Australia*, **152**, 565–66.

Craig, J.L. and Page, G. (1981) The questioning skills of nursing instructors. *Journal of Nursing Education*, **20**(5), 18–2.

Darbyshire, P., Stewart, B. and Jamieson, L. (1990) New domains in nursing. *Nursing Times*, **86**(27), 73–5.

Davis, A.R. (1988) Developing teaching strategies based on new knowledge. *Journal of Nursing Education*, **27**(4), 156–60.

Dennis, C. (1989) The nature of problems encountered in clinical practice: social support and stress levels of undergraduate nursing students. Unpublished report. School of Medical Education, University of New South Wales.

de Tornyay, R. (1982) *Strategies for Teaching Nursing*, John Wiley, New York.

Dewey, J. (1916) *Democracy and Education*. MacMillan, New York.

Dewey, J. (1938) *Experience and Education*, Macmillan, New York.

DiRienzo, J.N. (1983) Before client care – an interactive conference. *Journal of Nursing Education*, **22**(2), 84–6.

Dowling, C., Rotem, A. and White, R. (1982) Nurses and primary health care. Perceptions of nurses in New South Wales. Research and development monograph, WHO Regional Teacher Training Centre, University of New South Wales.

Duffy, B. (1986) Learning theories and the ward tutorial. *Nursing Education Today*, **6**, 23–7.

Duhamel, R. (1982) Administration: theory or practice. *Interchange on Educational Policy*, **13**, 2.

Elliott, R., Jillings, C. and Thorne, S. (1982) Psychomotor skill acquisition in nursing students in Canada and the U.S. *The Canadian Nurse*, **78**(3), 25–7.

Emden, C. (1988) Nursing knowledge: an intriguing journey. *The Australian Journal of Advanced Nursing*, **8**(2), 33–45.

Ewan, C. (1985) Curriculum Reform: has it missed its mark? *Medical Education*, **19**, 266–75.

Ewan, C. and White, R. (1984) *Teaching Nursing. A Self-Instructional Handbook*, Croom Helm, London.

Fawcett, J. (1983) Theory: basis for the study and practice of nursing education. *Journal of Nursing Education*, **24**(6), 226–43.

Fawcett, J. (1989) *Conceptual Models of Nursing*, 2nd ed., F.A. Davis Company, Philadelphia.

Field, W.E., Gallman, L., Nicholson, R. and Dreher, M. (1984) Clinical competencies of baccalaureate students. *Journal of Nursing Education*, **23**(7), 284–93.

Fishel, A.H. and Johnson, G.A. (1981) The three-way conference – nursing student, nursing supervisor and nursing educator. *Journal of Nursing Education*, **20**(6), 18–23.

Fitts, P.M. and Posner, M.L. (1967) *Human Performance*, Wadsworth, Belmont, CA.

Flagler, S., Loper-Powers, S. and Spitzer, A. (1988) Clinical teaching is more than evaluation alone! *Journal of Nursing Education*, **27**(8), 342–8.

Gagne, R.M. (1976) *Essentials of Learning for Instruction*, Dryden Press, Hinsdale, IL.

Gibbon, C. (1989) Contract learning in a clinical context: report of a case study. *Nurse Education Today*, **9**, 264–70.

Goldenberg, D. and Iwasiw, C. (1988) Criteria used for patient selection for nursing students' hospital clinical experience. *Journal of Nursing Education*, **27**(6), 258–65.

Goldhammer, R. (1969) *Clinical Supervision: Special Methods for the Supervision of Teachers*, Holt, Rinehart and Winston, New York.

Gomez, G.E. and Gomez, E.A. (1987) Learning of psychomotor skills: laboratory versus patient care setting. *Journal of Nursing Education*, **26**(1), 20–4.

Good, B.J. and Delvecchio Good, M.J. (1980) The meaning of symptoms: a cultural hermeneutic model for clinical practice. In: Eisenberg, L., Kleinman, A. (eds) *The relevance of social science for medicine*. Reidel, Boston, MA., pp. 165–96.

Greaves, F. (1979) Teaching nurses in clinical settings – 2. *Nursing Mirror Supplement*, 1 March, i–xii.

Guidelines for Curricula (1984) NSW Nurses Registration Board, Sydney, Australia.

Heath, T. (1979) Observation, Perception and Education. (1980) *Eur. Journal of Science Education*, **2**(7), 155–60.

Hedin, B. (1988) Expert clinical teaching, in *Curriculum Revolution: Reconceptualizing Nursing Education*, New York, National League for Nursing, Pub. No. 15-2280.

Hegarty-Hazel (1988) Prior learning challenges and critical thinking in the medical student laboratory in Cox, K. and Ewan, C. *The Medical Teacher*, Churchill Livingstone, London.

Henderson, V. (1966) *The Nature of Nursing*, Macmillan, New York.

Heron, J. (1977) *Dimensions of Facilitator Style*. University of Surrey, Guildford, pp. 3–20.

Higgs, J. (1982) A training programme for physiotherapy clinical supervisors. Unpublished Major Project, Master of Health Personnel Education Degree, School of Medical Education, University of New South Wales.

House, J.S. (1981) *Work Stress and Social Support*. Addison-Wesley. Reading, MA.

Infante, M.S. (1975) *The Clinical Laboratory in Nursing Education*, John Wiley, New York.

Infante, M.S. (1985) *The Clinical Laboratory in Nursing Education*, 2nd ed., John Wiley, New York.

Keller, J.M. (1983) Motivational design of instruction, in Riegeluth, C.M. (ed.) *Instructional-design Theories and Models: An Overview of their Present Status*, pp. 386–434, Lawrence Erlbaum, Hillsdale, NJ.

Kermode, S. (1985) Clinical supervision in nurse education: some parallels with teacher education. *The Australian Journal of Nursing*, **2**(3), 39–45.

Kermode, S. (1986) A conceptual framework for nursing practice. *The Australian Journal of Advanced Nursing*, **3**(3), 27–34.

Kermode, S. (1987) An exploratory study of students' use of the concepts on which a nursing curriculum is built. Unpublished Major Project, Master of Health Personnel Degree, School of Medical Education, University of New South Wales, Sydney.

Kieffer, J.S. (1984) Selecting technical skills to teach for competency. *Journal of Nursing Education*, **23**(5), 198–203.

Kim, H.S. (1983) *The Nature of Theoretical Thinking in Nursing*. Appleton-Century Crofts, Norwalk.

Kleehammer, K., Hart, A. and Keck, J. (1990) Nursing students' perceptions of anxiety-producing situations in the clinical setting, *Journal of Nursing Education*, **29**(4), 183–7.

Knowles, M. (1975) *Self-Directed Learning*. Follett Publishing, Chicago.

Kolb, D.A. (1984) *Experiential Learning: Experiences as the Source of Learning and Development*, Prentice-Hall, New Jersey.

Kramer, M. (1974) *Reality Shock: Why Nurses Leave Nursing*, C.V. Mosby, St Louis.

Karuhije, H.F. (1986) Preparation for clinical teaching. *Journal of Nursing Education*, **25**(4), 137–44.

Leininger, M. and Watson, J. (1990) *The Caring Imperative in Education*. Center for Human Caring. National League for Nursing, Pub No 41-2308.

Lindeman, C.A. (1989a) Curriculum revolution: reconceptualizing clinical nursing education. *Nursing and Health Care*, January, 23–8.

Lindeman, C.A. (1989b) Clinical teaching: paradoxes and paradigms, in *Curriculum Revolution. Reconceptualizing Nursing Education*. National League for Nursing, New York.

Little, P. and Ryan, G. (1988) Educational change through problem-based learning. *The Australian Journal of Advanced Nursing*, **5**(4), 31–5.

Lumby, J. (1987) Effective behaviours of clinical teachers. Unpublished Major Project, Master of Health Personnel Education Degree, School of Medical Education, University of New South Wales.

MacMillan, M.A. and Dwyer, J. (1989a) Changing times, changing paradigms (1): from hospital training and college education in Australia. *Nurse Education Today*, **9**(1), 13–18.

MacMillan, M.A. and Dwyer, J. (1989b) Changing times, changing paradigms (2): The Macarthur Experience. *Nurse Education Today*, **9**, 93–9.

McCoin, D.W. and Jenkins, P.C. (1988) Methods of assignment for pre-planning activities (advance student preparation) for the clinical experience. *Journal of Nursing Education*, **27**(2), 85–7.

McGaghie, W.C., Miller, G.E., Sajid, A.W. and Telder, T.V. (1978) Competency-based curriculum development in medical education: an introduction. Public Health Papers No. 68, Geneva, World Health Organization.

Marinker, M. (1974) Medical education and human values. *Journal of the Royal College of General Practitioners*, **24**, 445–62.

Marriner, A. (1986) *Nursing Theorists and their Work*, C.V. Mosby, St Louis.

Maslow, A.H. (1954) *Motivation and Personality*, Harper and Row, New York.

Mason, R.E. (1972) *Contemporary Educational Theory*, David McKay, New York.

Matheney, R.V. (1969) Pre- and post-clinical conferences for students. *American Journal of Nursing*, **69**(2), 286–9.

Meleca, C.B., Schimpfauser, F.T. and Witteman, J.K. (1978) *A Comprehensive and Systematic Assessment of Clinical Teaching Skills and Strategies in the Health Sciences*, US Department of Health, Education and Welfare, Public Health Service, National Institutes of Health.

Melia, K.M. (1984) Student nurses' construction of occupational socialisation. *Sociology of Health and Illness*, **6**, 133–51.

Mill, J. (1989) Linking theory to practice – developing a clinical practicum course for occupational therapy students. Unpublished Major Project, Master of Health Personnel Degree, School of Medical Education, University of New South Wales.

Mitchell, C.A. and Krainovich, B. (1982) Conducting pre- and post-conferences. *American Journal of Nursing*, May, 823–5.

Monjan, S.V. and Gassner, M. (1979) *Critical Issues in Competency-Based Education*, Pergamon Press, New York.

Montag, M. (1951) *The Education of Nursing Technicians*, John Wiley, New York.

Newman, M.A. (1979) *Theory Development in Nursing*, F.A. Davis, Philadelphia.

Norris, C. (1975) Restlessness: a nursing phenomenon insearch of meaning. *Nursing Outlook*, **23**, 103–7.

Novak, J.D. (1977) *A Theory of Education*, Cornell University Press, Ithaca.

Orlando, I.J. (1961) *The Dynamic Nurse-Patient Relationship*. G.P. Putnam, New York.

O'Shea, H.S. and Parsons, M.K. (1979) Clinical instruction: effective and ineffective teacher behaviours. *Nursing Outlook*, June, 411–15.

Pagana, K.D. (1988) Stresses and threats reported by baccalaureate students in relation to an initial clinical experience. *Journal of Nursing Education*, **279**, 418–24.

Partridge, B. (1989) The application of Orlando's theory of nursing. Unpublished Master's Thesis, Phillip Institute of Technology, Melbourne.

Pearson, M. and Smith, D. (1985) Debriefing in experience-based learning, in Boud *et al.* (eds) *Reflection: Turning Experience into Learning*, Kogan Page, London.

Phenix, P. (1964) *Realms of Meaning*, McGraw Hill, New York.

Posner, G.J. (1985) *Field Experience. A Guide to Reflective Teaching*, Longman, New York.

Powell, A. (1988) Learning by nursing students in the clinical setting: the influence of the qualified practitioner. Master of Education (Long Essay), University of Sydney.

Pratt, R. (1989) Sine qua non: the psychomotor skills profile of beginning practitioners in nursing. Major Project, Master of Health Personnel Degree, School of Medical Education, University of New South Wales.

Putt, A. (1978) *General Systems Theory Applied to Nursing*. Little, Brown, Boston.

Reigeluth, C.M. (ed.) (1983) *Instructional Design Theories and Models. An Overview of their Current Status*. Lawrence Erlbaum, Hillsdale, NJ.

Reihl, J.P. and Roy, C. (1980) *Conceptual Models for Nursing Practice*. Appleton-Century Crofts, New York.

Reilly, D.E. (1990) Research in nursing education. Yesterday-today-tomorrow. *Nursing and Health Care*, March, 139–43.

Reilly, D.E. and Oermann, M.H. (1985) *The Clinical Field. Its Use in Nursing Education*, Appleton-Century Crofts, Norwalk.

Retallick, J. (1986) Clinical supervision: technical, collaboration and critical approaches, in Smyth, J. (ed.) (1986) *Learning About Teaching Through Clinical Supervision*, Croom Helm, Sydney.

Ritchie, J. (1986) Development of a model to assist health professionals in supporting patients to assume self-responsibility. Unpublished Major Project, Master of Health Personnel Degree. School of Medical Education. University of New South Wales.

Rogers, C. (1969) *Freedom to Learn*, Charles E. Merrill, Columbus, OH.

Rogers, C. (1983) *Freedom to Learn for the 80's*, Charles E. Merrill, Columbus, OH.

Romanini, J. (1988) A teaching management model for interactive learning. Major Project, Master of Health Personnel Degree, School of Medical Education, University of New South Wales, Sydney.

Roper, N. (1980) *The Elements of Nursing*, Churchill Livingstone, Edinburgh.

Roper, N., Logan, W. and Tierney, A. (1983) *Using a Model for Nursing*, Churchill Livingstone, London.

Roy, Sr. C. (1970) Adaptation: a conceptual framework for nursing, *Nursing Outlook*, **18**, 3.

Russell, R.L. (1980) Conceptual models for teaching: a current examination. *The Australian Nurses Journal*, **10**(2), 38–42.

Ryan, G. (1989) Problem-based learning – some practical issues. *Research and Development in Higher Education*, **11**, 155–9.

Ryan, G. and Little, P. (1989) Problem-based learning within the School of Nursing and Health Studies at Macarthur Institute of Higher Education, in Wallis, B. (ed.) *Problem-Based Learning – The Newcastle Workshop*, Faculty of Medicine, University of Newcastle.

Salisbury, D.F., Richards, B.F. and Klein, J.D. (1985) Designing practice: a review of prescriptions and recommendations from instructional design theories. *Journal of Instructional Development*, **8**(4), 9–19.

Sando, J. (1989) Interpersonal skills for nurses. Unpublished Major Project, Master of Health Personnel Degree, School of Medical Education, University of New South Wales.

Sasmor, J.L. (1984) Contracting for clinical. *Journal of Nursing Education*, **23**(4), 171–3.

Schon, D.A. (1988) *Educating the Reflective Practitioner*, Jossey-Bass, San Francisco.

Schweer, J.E. (1972) *Creative Teaching in Clinical Nursing*, 2nd ed., C.V. Mosby, St Louis.

Sergiovanni, T. (1986) A theory of practice for clinical supervision, in Smyth J. (ed.) *Learning about Teaching Through Clinical Supervision*, Croom Helm, Sydney.

Silver, M. (1989) Career structure for nurses: the South Australian experience. In, Gray G. and Pratt R. (eds) (1989) *Issues in Australian Nursing 2*, Churchill Livingstone, Melbourne.

Simpson, I.H. (1979) *From Student to Nurse*, Cambridge University Press, Cambridge.

Singer, R.N. (1980) *Motor Learning and Human Performance*, McMillan Publishing Company, New York.

Skurski, V. (1985) Interactive clinical conferences: nursing rounds and educational imagery. *Journal of Nursing Education*, **24**(4), 166–8.

Smyth, W.J. (1984) *Clinical Supervision-Collaborative Learning about Teaching, A Handbook*, Deakin University Press, Victoria.

Smyth, W.J. (ed.) (1986) *Learning about Teaching through Clinical Supervision*, Croom Helm, London.

Smythe, E. (1984) *Surviving Nursing*, Addison-Wesley, Reading, MA.

Stein, H.F. (1984) The ethnographic mode of teaching clinical behavioural science, in Chrisman, N.J., Maretzki, T.W. (eds) *Clinically applied Anthropology*, Reidel, Boston, MA.

Stevens, B.J. (1979) *Nursing Theory. Analysis, Application, Evaluation.* Little and Brown. Boston.

Storch, J.L. (1986) In defence of nursing theory. *The Canadian Nurse,* January, 16–20.

Sweeney, M.A., Hedstrom, B. and O'Malley, M. (1982) Process Evaluation: A second look at psychomotor skills. *Journal of Nursing Education,* **21**(2), 4–17.

Swendsen-Boss, L. (1985) Teaching for clinical competence. *Nurse Educator,* **10**(4), 8–12.

Tan, L. (1987) Implementing holistic conceptual framework in psychomotor nursing skills. Unpublished Major Project, Master of Health Personnel Degree, School of Medical Education, University of New South Wales.

Tanner, C.A. and Lindeman, C.A. (1987) Research in nursing education: Assumptions and priorities. *Journal of Nursing Education,* **26**, 50–60.

Taylor, J.A. and Cleveland, P.J. (1984) Effective use of the learning laboratory. *Journal of Nursing Education,* **23**(1), 32–4.

Thompson, D.G. and Williams, R.G. (1985) Barriers to the acceptance of problem-based learning in medical schools. *Studies in Higher Education,* **2**(1), 79–119.

Townsend, J. (1990a) Problem-based learning. *Nursing Times,* **86**(4), 61–2.

Townsend, J. (1990b) Teaching/learning strategies. *Nursing Times,* **86**(23), 66–8.

Turkoski, B. (1987) Reducing stress in nursing students' clinical learning experience. *Journal of Nursing Education,* **26**(8), 335–7.

Turney, C., Cairns, L., Williams, G., Hatton, N. and Owens, L. (1973) *Sydney Micro Skills,* Series 1 Handbook, Sydney University Press, Sydney.

Turney, C., Cairns, L., Williams, G., Hatton, N. and Owens, L. (1975) *Sydney Micro Skills,* Series 2 Handbook, Sydney University Press, Sydney.

Turney, C., Cairns, L., Eltis, K., Hatton, N., Thew, D., Towler, J. and Wright, R. (1982) *Supervisor Development Programmes,* Role Handbook, Sydney University Press, Sydney.

Watts, N. (1990) *Handbook of Clinical Teaching,* Churchill Livingstone, Melbourne.

Werner-McCullough, M. and l'Orange, C. (1985) Putting oomph into clinical conferences. *Nurse Educator,* **10**(6), 33–5.

White, R., Ewan, C., Hatton, N., Higgs, J., Hickey, C. and Baker, K. (1988a) *Microskills for Clinical Teachers.* An instructional manual to accompany the videotapes *Positive Practices: Teaching Strategies for Nurse Educators* and *Teaching Practices: Teaching Strategies for Medical, Nursing and Therapy Educators,* School of Medical Education, University of New South Wales.

White, R., Ewan, C., Hatton, N. and Lovitt, L. (1988b) *Critical Incidents in Clinical Teaching.* Perspectives from the Social and Behavioural Sciences. An Instructional Manual for Nurse Educators, School of Medical Education, University of New South Wales.

Windows onto Worlds (1987) *Studying Australia at Tertiary Level*, AGPS, Canberra.

Windsor, A. (1987) Nursing students' perceptions of clinical experience. *Journal of Nursing Education*, **26**(4), 150–4.

FURTHER READING

Andrusyszyn, M.A. (1989) Clinical evaluation of the affective domain. *Nurse Education Today*, **9**, 75–81.

Arendt, H. (1971) *The Life of the Mind*. Vol. 1, *Thinking*. Harcourt Brace Jovanovich. San Diego, CA.

Barnett, R.A., Becher, R.A. and Cork, N.M. (1987) Models of professional preparation: pharmacy, nursing and teacher education. *Studies in Higher Education*, **12**(1), 51–63.

Barrows, H.S. (1985) *How to Design a Problem-Based Curriculum for the Pre-clinical Years*, Springer, New York.

Barrows, H.S. (1986) A taxonomy of problem-based learning methods. *Medical Education*, **20**(6), 481–6.

Barrows, H.S. and Tamblyn, R.M. (1980) *Problem-based Learning: An Approach to Medical Education*. Springer, New York.

Bawden, R. (1985) Problem-based learning: an Australian perspective, in Boud, C. (ed.) *Problem-Based Learning in Education for the Professions*. HERDSA, Sydney.

Boud, D. (ed.) (1981) *Developing Student Autonomy in Learning*, Kogan Page, London.

Boud, D., Dunn, J., Kennedy, T. and Walker, M. (1978) *Laboratory Teaching in Tertiary Science*, Higher Education Research and Development Society of Australia (HERDSA), Sydney.

Brittain, J.N. Spiritual care: integration into a collegiate nursing curriculum. *Journal of Nursing Education*, **26**(4), 155–60.

Burnard, P. (1989) Developing critical ability in nurse education. *Nurse Education Today*, **9**, 271–5.

Carroll, E. (1988) The role of tacit knowledge in problem solving in the clinical setting. *Nurse Education Today*, **9**, 140–7.

Carter, R. (1985) A taxonomy of objectives for professional education. *Studies in Higher Education*, **10**(2), 135–49.

Condell, S.L. and Elliott, N. (1989) Gagne's theory of instruction – its relevance to nurse education. *Nurse Education Today*, **9**, 281–4.

Cox, K.R. (1987) Knowledge which cannot be used is useless. *Medical Teacher*, **9**(2), 145–54.

Davidhizar, R.W. and McBride, A. (1985) How nursing students explain their success and failure in clinical experiences. *Journal of Nursing Education*, **24**(7), 284–90.

Dowie, S. and Park, C. (1988) Relating nursing theory to students' life experiences. *Nurse Education Today*, **8**, 191–6.

Fong, C. (1990) Role overload, social support and burnout among nursing educators. *Journal of Nursing Education*, **29**(3), 102–8.
Frey, L. and Reigeluth, C.M. (1986) Instructional models for tutoring: a review. *Journal of Instructional Development*, **9**(1), 2–8.
Gagne, R.M. (1985) *The Conditions of Learning*, 4th ed., Holt, Rinehart and Winston, New York.
Garman, N.B. (1986) Getting to the essence of practice in clinical supervision, in Smyth, W.J. (ed.) *Learning about Teaching through Clinical Supervision*, Croom Helm, London.
Gates, R.J. (1989) Teacher behaviour: a determinant of student self esteem. *Nurse Education Today*, **9**, 207–10.
Gerace, L. and Sibilano, H. (1984) Preparing students for peer collaboration: a clinical teaching model. *Journal of Nursing Education*, **23**(5), 206–9.
Gray, G. and Pratt, R. (eds) (1989) *Issues in Australian Nursing 2*, Churchill Livingstone, Melbourne.
Hall, E. (1961) *Silent Language*. New York, Premier Books.
Hart, G. (1990) Peer consultation and review. *The Australian Journal of Advanced Nursing*, **7**(2), 40–6.
Hegarty, E.H. (1979) How to organize effective laboratory teaching in medicine. Part 1. Purposes. *Medical Teacher*, **1**(4), 175–81.
Hegarty, E.H. (1982) Teaching in the laboratory, in Cox, K.R. and Ewan, C.E. (ed.) *The Medical Teacher*, Churchill Livingstone, London.
Hentinen, M. (1985) A programme for developing nurses' skills and nursing practice. *Journal of Advanced Nursing*, **10**, 405–16.
Hepworth, S. (1989) Professional judgement and nurse education. *Nurse Education Today*, **9**, 408–12.
Iwasiw, C. (1987) The role of the teacher in self-directed learning. *Nurse Education Today*, **7**, 222–7.
Jarvis, P. (1983) *Professional Education*, Croom Helm, Beckenham.
Jones, C. (1983) Negotiating student placements in ambulatory settings. *Journal of Nursing Education*, **22**(6), 255–8.
Kermode, S. (1988) How nurses use curriculum concepts. *Australian Journal of Advanced Nursing*, **6**(1), 21–6.
King, I.M. (1981) *A Theory for Nursing. Systems, concepts, process*. John Wiley, New York.
Knowles, M. (1986) *The Adult Learner: a Neglected Species*, 3rd ed., Gulf Publishing Company, Houston.
Levine, M.E. (1973) *Introduction to Clinical Nursing*, 2nd ed., F.A. Davis, Philadelphia.
Lewis, K.E. and Tamblyn, R.M. (1987) The problem-based learning approach in baccalaureate nursing education: how effective is it? *Nursing Papers/Perspectives in Nursing*, **19**(2), 17–26.
Locasto, L. and Kochanek, D. (1989) Reality shock in the nurse educator. *Journal of Nursing Education*, **28**(2), 79–81.
Marsick, V.J. (ed.) (1987) *Learning in the Workplace*. Croom Helm, London.
Marton, R. and Saljo, R. (1976) Qualitative differences in learning outcome

as a function of the learner's conception of the task. *British Journal of Educational Psychology*, **46**, 115–27.

Mead, M. (1955) *Cultural Patterns and Cultural Change*, Menton, New York.

Megel, M.E., Wilken, M.K. and Volcek, M.K. (1987) Nursing students' performance: Administering injections in laboratory and clinical area. *Journal of Nursing Education*, **26**(7), 288–93.

Meyers, C. (1986) *Teaching Students to Think Critically*, Jossey-Bass, London.

Miller, A. (1985) The relationship between nursing theory and nursing practice. *Journal of Advanced Nursing*, **10**, 411–24.

Mogan, J. and Thorne, S. (1985) Injection giving: the effect of time lapse between learning and actual practice on student confidence. *Nursing Papers*, **17**(2), 49–58.

Neuman, B. (1982) *The Neuman Systems Model. Application to Nursing Education and Practice*. Appleton-Century Crofts, Norwalk.

Novak, J.D. (1979) Improvement of laboratory teaching, *The American Biology Teacher*, **41**, 467–470.

Novak, J.D. (1985) Application of advances in learning theory and philosophy of science to the improvement of higher education. HERDSA.

Olson, R.K., Gresley, R.S. and Heater, B.S. (1984) The effects of undergraduate internship on the self-concept and professional role mastery of baccalaureate nursing students. *Journal of Nursing Education*, **23**(3), 105–8.

Perry, W.G. (1970) *Forms of Intellectual and Ethical Development in the College Years*, Holt, Rinehart and Winston, New York.

Pratt, R. (1989) Sine Qua Non: The Psychomotor Skills Profile of Beginning Practitioners in Nursing. Unpublished master degree major project. School of Medical Education, University of New South Wales, Sydney.

Pugh, E. (1986) Use of behavioural observation to augment quantitative data when studying clinical teaching. *Journal of Nursing Education*, **25**(8), 341–3.

Rajek, N.J. (1987) Developing an evening clinical experience for baccalaureate community health nursing students, *Journal of Nursing Education*, **26**(5), 197–200.

Ramsden, P. (1979) Student learning and perceptions of the academic environment. *Higher Education*, **8**, 411–27.

Reilly, D.E. (1989) Ethics and values in nursing: are we opening Pandora's Box? *Nursing and Health Care*, February, 91–5.

Robertson, C.M. (1980) *Clinical Teaching*. Pitman Books, London.

Rodgers, B.L. and Cowles, K.V. (1990) The advanced practicum project. *Nursing Outlook*, **38**(1), 31–5.

Rogers, M.E. (1970) *An Introduction to the Theoretical Basis of Nursing*, F.A. Davis, Philadelphia.

Ryan, M. (1985) Assimilating the learning needs of RN students into the clinical practicum. *Journal of Nursing Education*, **24**(3), 128–30.

Schoolcraft, V. and Delaney, C. (1982) Contract grading in clinical evaluation. *Journal of Nursing Education*, **21**(1), 6–14.

Sheahan, J. (1980) Educating teachers of nursing: a survey of the opinions of students. *Journal of Advanced Nursing*, **5**(1), 71–81.

Sheahan, J. (1982) Educating teachers of nursing: the attitudes of students. *Journal of Advanced Nursing*, **7**(1), 69–77.

Smith, D.W. (1968) *Perspectives on Clinical Teaching*. Springer, New York.

Smithers, K. and Bircumshaw, D. (1988) The student experience of undergraduate education: the relationship between academic and clinical learning environments. *Nurse Education Today*, **8**(6), 347–53.

Wallis, B. (ed.) (1989) *Problem-based Learning – The Newcastle Workshop*, Faculty of Medicine, University of Newcastle.

Whitis, G. (1985) Simulation in teaching clinical nursing. *Journal of Nursing Education*, **24**(4), 161–3.

Witkin, H.A., Moore, C.A., Goodenough, D.R. and Cox, P.W. (1977) Field-dependent and field-independent cognitive styles and their educational implications. *Review of Educational Research*, **47**, 1–64.

Wong, J. (1979) The inability to transfer classroom learning to clinical nursing practice: a learning problem and its remedial plan. *Journal of Advanced Nursing*, **4**, 161–8.

Wong, S. (1978) Nursing-teacher behaviours in the clinical field: apparent effect on nursing students' learning. *Journal of Advanced Nursing*, **3**, 369–72.

Wong, S. and Wong, J. (1980) The effectiveness of clinical teaching: a model for self-evaluation. *Journal of Advanced Nursing*, **5**(5), 531–7.

Yonke, A.M. (1979) The art and science of clinical teaching. *Medical Education*, **13**, 86–90.

Index

GPSR Compliance
The European Union's (EU) General Product Safety Regulation (GPSR) is a set of rules that requires consumer products to be safe and our obligations to ensure this.

If you have any concerns about our products, you can contact us on

ProductSafety@springernature.com

In case Publisher is established outside the EU, the EU authorized representative is:

Springer Nature Customer Service Center GmbH
Europaplatz 3
69115 Heidelberg, Germany

www.ingramcontent.com/pod-product-compliance
Ingram Content Group UK Ltd.
Pitfield, Milton Keynes, MK11 3LW, UK
UKHW040704051126
16351UKWH00008B/36
* 9 7 8 1 4 8 9 9 3 3 5 5 3 *